Community Health Nurs...

Primary Health Care in Practice

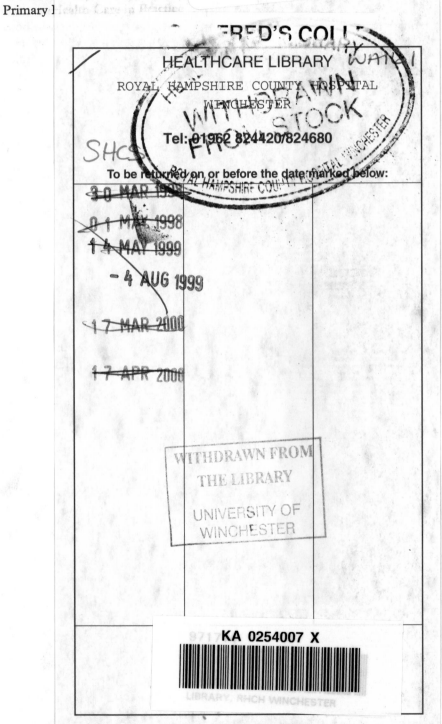

Anne McMurray RN PhD FRCNA

Anne McMurray's nursing education began in Canada and she has practised in community health, occupational health and health promotion in both Canada and Australia. She has also taught nursing in both countries. Her present appointment is Professor, and Head of School of Nursing, Edith Cowan University, Perth, WA.

For Churchill Livingstone in Melbourne
Publisher: Judy Waters
Editorial: Maja Ingrassia
Desktop Preparation: Sandra Tolra
Indexing: Max McMaster
Production Controller: Peter Hylands
Design: Jan Schmoeger

Community Health Nursing
Primary Health Care in Practice

Second Edition

Anne McMurray RN PhD FRCNA

CHURCHILL LIVINGSTONE
MELBOURNE EDINBURGH LONDON MADRID NEW YORK TOKYO 1993

CHURCHILL LIVINGSTONE
Medical Division of Longman Group UK Limited

Distributed in Australia by Longman Australia Pty Limited, Longman House, Kings Gardens, 95 Coventry Street, South Melbourne 3205, and by associated companies, branches and representatives throughout the world.

© Longman Group UK Limited 1993
except for material listed on pp. vii and viii

First edition 1990
Second edition 1993
   Reprinted 1994
   Reprinted 1995

National Library of Australia Cataloguing in Publication Data

McMurray, Anne.
   Community health nursing.
   2nd ed.
   ISBN 0443 04865 7.

   1. Community health nursing. 2. Community health services. I. Title.

610.7343

The publisher's policy is to use paper manufactured from sustainable forests

Produced by Churchill Livingstone in Melbourne
Printed in Malaysia — VVP

Acknowledgements

This work is testimony to the process of collegial communication. I am grateful to my students, colleagues and friends for providing me with feedback on the first edition of the book so that the second edition would be relevant to both teaching and learning needs. In particular, I would like to thank those nurses in urban, rural and remote Australian communities who have been kind enough to share the wisdom and insight of their experiences and, once again, I would like to thank Judy Waters for her invaluable assistance in preparing the manuscript.

A.M.

For my parents

Copyright acknowledgements

CHAPTER 3
Fig. 3.1 The Neuman health care systems model. From: Benedict M, Behringer Sproles J 1987 Application of the Neuman model to public health nursing practice. In: Neuman B (ed) The Neuman systems model. Appleton-Century-Crofts, Norwalk, CT, USA.

Fig. 3.3 Pender's health promotion model. From: Pender N 1987 Health promotion in nursing practice, 2nd edn. Appleton & Lange, Norwalk, CT, USA.

CHAPTER 4
Fig. 4.1 A comparison of Maslow's identification of basic needs of the individual with those of the community as client. From: Higgs G, Gustafson D 1985 Community as a client: assessment and diagnosis. F A Davis, Vancouver, BC.

CHAPTER 6
Fig. 6.2 Blank genogram. From: Wright L, Leahey M 1984 Nurses and families: a guide to family assessment and intervention. F A Davis, Vancouver, BC.

Fig. 6.3 Symbols used in genograms. From: Wright L, Leahey M 1984 Nurses and families: a guide to family assessment and intervention. F A Davis, Vancouver, BC.

CHAPTER 7
Fig. 7.1 The PRECEDE-PROCEED model for health promotion planning and evaluation. From: *Health Education Planning: A Diagnostic Approach* by Green et al. By permission of Mayfield Publishing Company. Copyright © 1980 by Mayfield Publishing Company.

APPENDIX 1
Standards for community nursing practice. From: Australian Council of Community Nursing Services 1993 Australian Council of Community Nursing Services Standards for community nursing practice. ACCNS, Melbourne.

APPENDIX 2

The Friedman family assessment model (short form). From: Friedman M 1992 Family nursing: theory and practice, 3rd edn. Appleton & Lange, Norwalk, CT, USA.

APPENDIX 3

Community assessment tool. From: Clark MJD 1984 Community nursing: health care for today and tomorrow, Appendix C. Appleton-Century-Crofts, Norwalk, CT, USA.

Contents

Preface

'Community' is, for most people, a friendly term. It conjures up a sense of place, a sense of belonging. A healthy community is one in which belonging is valued, where the connections between individuals, families and the environment are as important as the life forces within. A healthy community is thus a caring community.

As the next century approaches, the need for a caring community becomes even more acute than in the past. Individual victims of political and economic circumstances need to be cared for. Families, in particular, need a caring environment in which to either maintain themselves or adapt to changing structural, social and financial conditions. Environmental issues, such as overpopulation, land degradation, global warming and pollution dictate that we must all develop a caring approach to our social and physical community, reconsidering our community membership in terms of the wider global community.

This book is intended to challenge nurses to nurture caring in the community. It is a plea to nurses in all communities to adopt the primary health care principles of equity, access, empowerment, cultural sensitivity and self-determinism to mediate, educate and facilitate environmentally friendly health care for the community and the individuals and families who live there.

Those familiar with the first edition will notice that some parts have been rearranged, others omitted and some new material added. In the new edition, the Ottawa Charter for Health Promotion is emphasized as a strategic framework for planning primary health care activities in the community. In addition, a number of case studies based on research findings from the author's study on expertise in community health nursing are included. This book also expands on the first edition by including broader discussion on such topics as Aboriginal health and family nursing. The final chapter accentuates the theme that community health nurses must be responsive to the community they serve, and provides an indepth discussion of five major trends and issues which will affect practice as we move towards the next century. These include the environment, the changing face of the community, AIDS and its impact on society, ethical issues in primary health care and the evolving role of the nurse. It is my intention that this not be a static list of trends and issues, but a point of provocation for ongoing dialogue on the physical, social and political context in which nursing is practised.

Since the first edition was published many nurses throughout Australia and elsewhere have provided comments and suggestions which have been incorporated into this text. If the book has no effect beyond acting as a stimulus for this type of sharing I will consider it a success. It is offered in the spirit of our collegial goal of helping to achieve health for all communities.

PART 1

The community health nurse

INTRODUCTION

Community health nursing is much more than nursing practised in the community. It is a unique and continually evolving specialized area within the profession of nursing which considers the *context* of people's lives as paramount to attaining and maintaining health. Community health nurses practise in a wide variety of settings, each with unique characteristics which impact on practice goals and strategies, yet each of which are connected to the other through the common philosophy of primary health care. By aspiring to the holistic and comprehensive primary health care goal of health for all, nurses can facilitate and enable people in communities everywhere to secure a healthful and productive life. This section addresses the fundamental concepts and issues related to practising community health nursing within the framework of primary health care. Chapter 1 provides an overview of common themes and goals shared by all community health nurses, while Chapter 2 provides examples of the variety of roles adopted by nurses working with different types of communities. It is hoped that these first two chapters will initiate a dialogue on how best to help communities to achieve their desired levels of health and to deal with ill health in a way that least compromises the quality of their lives.

Content: Part 1

1. Community health nursing and primary health care

Health, community health, and community health nursing
    Health
    Community health
    Community health nursing
Primary health care
    Principles of primary health care
        Equity
        Access
        Empowerment
        Cultural sensitivity
        Self-determinism
Primary health care as organizational strategy
The role of the community health nurse
Community health nursing compared to institutional nursing

2. Community health nursing specialties

Specialization
The specialist community health nurse
Developing a specialized role
    Role identification
    Role transition
    Role confirmation
Child health nursing
Community mental health nursing
School health nursing
Occupational health nursing
Remote area nursing

1. Community health nursing and primary health care

The health of a community is a multifaceted, dynamic, and challenging concern. The many facets include the historical, cultural, organizational, environmental and situational aspects of a community combined with the individual and collective needs, goals and aspirations of its population. The relative state of a community's health is dynamic, in that the combinations of these individual and situational characteristics are continually shifting and changing. The challenge for anyone concerned with community health lies in the process of becoming familiar with a community, discovering its uniqueness, learning what its particular needs and concerns are, and enabling and nurturing change or the maintenance of health. This is the challenge of community health nursing.

HEALTH, COMMUNITY HEALTH, AND COMMUNITY HEALTH NURSING

Health

Health can be defined in many ways. The World Health Organization has described 'health' as 'a state of complete physical, mental and social well being and not merely the absence of disease or infirmity' (WHO 1974, p. 1). This definition is useful in that it moves towards an holistic view of health, that is, one which encompasses physical, mental and social factors. However, it does not account for the broad variability in an individual's state of health, nor the way in which a person's view of health changes with time and circumstances.

Halfdan Mahler, the former Director General of WHO (1979), suggests that any useful definition of health must contain two key dimensions: health balance (or stability) and health potential. Maslow (1943) explains health potential in terms of self-actualization. He views health as reaching a stage where basic physical, social and emotional needs are met and where one is able to reach an extended state of well being (self-actualization) which allows free, spontaneous and creative behaviours to occur. However, Lawler (1983, 1991) challenges Maslow's model which suggests that self-actualization follows a predetermined sequence of hierarchical stages of

3

need fulfilment. According to Maslow (1943), the individual progresses from seeking to have basic needs (air, water, food) met, then safety needs, belongingness and love needs, esteem needs and ultimately, the need for self-actualization. Lawler (1991, p. 218) contends that such a prescriptive model may not be generalizeable given that 'the concept of need is influenced by such complex issues as class, culture, gender, age, language, values, education and economic reality, among other things'. In her view, the importance of one or another type of need is determined by the individual within the context of her or his culture and circumstances. Health and an individual's hierarchy of needs are thus culturally and socially determined.

Pender (1987) has proposed a definition of health which includes both health potential and health balance. She defines health as 'the actualization of inherent and acquired human potential through goal directed behaviour, competent self-care, and satisfying relationships with others while adjustments are made as needed to maintain structural integrity and harmony with the environment' (p. 27). Pender's definition reflects health as a process of development characterized by frequent experiences of challenge, achievement and satisfaction. She views health in the context of both internal and external environments. However, achieving and maintaining health is often compromised by these very environments. The physical, social and cultural environment often determines the extent to which health potential may be achieved. Indeed, the cultural environment may determine whether the individual wishes to pursue his or her potential for varying levels or states of health. For this reason, one must define health with caution, perhaps confining a global definition to the following:

Health is a state of equilibrium which derives from a balance between the striving for a self-determined state of well being and the compromises demanded by the physical, psychological, social and cultural environment.

Community health

Individual perceptions of health and health priorities (physical, emotional, social, spiritual) are bound to communal environments. Hudson-Rodd (1991) views health as an expression of life within specific environments. She suggests that 'in order to understand health, an awareness of the dynamic connection between a people and their environment is needed' (p. 1). This territorial identification is what Buttimer (1976) calls a 'sense of place'. Shotter (1985) suggests that it is a 'social space full of the enabling constraints offered us by the other people we meet in it. And such a space changes as we act in it' (p. 459).

A person's sense of place within a community is central to understanding how health is achieved and maintained, and how illness is overcome. Hudson-Rodd (1991) explains: 'Because they are expressions of culture, health, illness, and health care need to be understood in relation to each other. To examine one in isolation from each other distorts the knowledge of the nature of each and how they relate to one another' (p. 4). Individual health and community health are thus interdependent notions. As Shotter (1985) suggests, 'the self develops out of a human community...the understanding that individuals have of themselves will influence how they interact with their place' (p. 65). The individual cannot, therefore, achieve a state of equilibrium unless it is within a community context.

Clark (1984) defines a community as 'a group of people between whom there is some type of bond, who engage in interaction with each other, and who function collectively in regard to common concerns' (p. 5). From this perspective, any definition of community health must relate health to the aggregate or group context, including the idea of collective action with regard to common concerns. In addition, the bond between individual members, whether geographic or cultural, must be recognized. Finally, some type of human relationship or social interaction must be present (Clark 1984).

Clark's definition of the community as an interactive collective is aligned with the Goeppinger et al (1982) concept of community competence. If community health is seen as a process involving the health capabilities and potential for interaction within and external to the community, it is by definition, community competence (Goeppinger et al 1982). Eng et al (1992, p. 4) extend this notion, describing the community as a 'living organism with interactive webs of ties among organizations, neighbourhoods, families and friends'.

A further element in community health concerns the balance between individual and group goals and interactions. Efforts to achieve individual and community competence must be considered and negotiated within the constraints of the physical, psychological, cultural and social environment. A useful definition of community health may thus be as follows:

> Community health is a state of equilibrium which derives from a balance between the individual and collective striving for self-determined (and self-defined) well being, and the compromises demanded by the physical, psychological, cultural and social environment.

The two key dimensions of health—health balance and health potential—remain relevant for the individual, family, group and community.

Community health nursing

Community health nursing is much more than nursing practised in the community setting. It is the practice of simultaneously considering and enabling the health care needs of individuals, families, aggregates (population subgroups), and the total community. This demands both a clinical and public health focus of care (Williams 1986). Guided by the humanitarian ethos of respect for *all* people, the nurse attempts to intervene with individuals and families in ways that are culturally considerate, humanely committed and responsive (Salmon et al 1988). At the same time, the health needs of various subgroups and the collective needs of the population must also be considered. Additionally, community health nursing must be based on an ecological view of health. In other words, there must be ongoing consideration of the influence of environmental factors (physical, biological and sociocultural) on health and the interrelationships between the person and her or his environment (WHO Commission on Health and Environment 1992). This view of health is actually an extension of that proposed by Florence Nightingale. Nursing, she claimed, 'ought to signify the proper use of fresh air, light, warmth, cleanliness, quiet, and the proper selection and administration of diet—all at the least expense of the vital power to the patient' (Nightingale 1859, p. 6).

In Nightingale's day, caring and helping interventions were directed towards alleviating the pain and suffering of the war-wounded. Today, the caring and helping characteristics remain, but the role has gradually been extended and expanded so that care is provided and co-ordinated from a greatly increased and diversified knowledge base. The focus of nursing has shifted from paternalistic care-giving towards comprehensive, holistic and client-centred practice. It is comprehensive insofar as the nurse must be capable of practising on three levels of prevention: primary, for health promotion and protection from harm; secondary for care-giving and client advocacy; and tertiary, for restoration and rehabilitation once illness has occurred (see Fig. 1.1). The focus is holistic in that care is organized around the client in his or her entire or 'whole' context or environment. It is client-

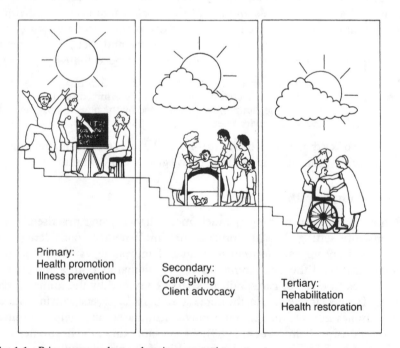

Primary:
Health promotion
Illness prevention

Secondary:
Care-giving
Client advocacy

Tertiary:
Rehabilitation
Health restoration

Fig. 1.1   Primary, secondary and tertiary prevention.

centred in that it is a collaborative effort between nurse and client to promote self-determined care and empowerment rather than dependence. In short, nursing the community is guided by the principles of primary health care.

PRIMARY HEALTH CARE

The ambitious social goal of the World Health Organization (WHO) and its member states is that the world achieve health for all by the year 2000. Maglacas (1988) explains that this commitment to health for all is not a cry for global eradication of disease or infirmity, but a pledge to consider health in the broader context of social and economic development; an attempt to secure socially and economically satisfying lives for all people. Dr Eric Goon, Director General of WHO, contends that health for all by the year 2000 is really an attempt to ensure that by that time, everybody has equitable access to health care services (Little 1992).

The nursing profession, through the International Council of Nurses (ICN), has declared its commitment to the goal of health for all by the year 2000 through primary health care (ICN-WHO 1979), a goal which is shared by the Australian Nursing Federation (ANF 1990). It is expected that nurses, as a unified force in primary health care, can effect positive changes in the health system to correct deficiencies and enable all people of the world to attain a healthful productive life (Morrow 1988).

Primary health care is explained in the Declaration of Alma Ata, a statement of commitment which was devised by delegates from 132 nations at Alma Ata in the former USSR, who met to consider how health for all people could be achieved. Primary health care was thus declared as:

Essential health care based on practical, scientifically sound and socially acceptable methods and technology made universally accessible to individuals and families in the community through their full participation and at a cost that the community and country can afford to maintain at every stage of their develop-ment in the spirit of self-reliance and self-determination. It is the first level of contact with individuals, the family and community with the national health systems bringing health care as close as possible to where people live and work, and constitutes the first element of a continuing health care process.

(WHO UNICEF 1978, p. 6)

Primary health care is therefore a *philosophy* permeating the entire health system, a *strategy* for organizing health care, a *level of care*, and a *set of activities* (Chamberlain & Beckingham 1987). Holzemer (1992) explains that the primary health care philosophy conceptualizes health as a fundamental right, an individual and collective responsibility, an equal opportunity concept and an essential element of socioeconomic development. As a level of care it is primary, that is, the first line of entry to the health care system, but broader than what is called primary care (initial care) in that primary health care also encompasses the collaborative activities of government, other sectors of society and the community itself (Smith et al 1985). This intersectoral involvement means that housing, population control and technology transfer, for example, should all be considered as instrumental in achieving health (Leeder & Grossman 1991). Primary health care must also be distinguished from primary nursing, which refers to a system for delivering nursing care in which one nurse has primary responsibility for planning, co-ordinating and evaluating the nursing care of a specific client or group of clients. As a set of activities, primary health care consists of those actions which implement the strategies for achieving health in the global as well as local community.

Principles of primary health care

The philosophy of primary health care revolves around the principles of equity, access, empowerment, cultural sensitivity and self-determinism. These five principles provide an important framework for nursing practice in the community.

Equity

An equitable system of health care is one in which all members of society have equal opportunity to achieve health. Equity in health care has thus far been difficult to achieve. Indeed, we have not as yet been able to secure health for the majority of the world's citizens, particularly for those most vulnerable to ill health. Seven million children die every year of diarrhoea which could be prevented by the provision of safe drinking water (WHO 1989). Many families throughout the world live in poverty. In Australia, approximately 360 000 children were living in families with incomes below the poverty line in 1988. This represents 10% of the nation's children (McDonald 1990). In both developed and developing countries, the cost of health care continues to escalate, subordinating equity to economic arrangements. In the developing nations the problem is primarily a lack of resources. In the developed countries it is the inequitable distribution of health care within over-bureaucratized health care structures. Cuthbert (1989) cites data from the Australian Institute of Health (AIH) which identifies those with lower education and income as being at higher than average risk for acute and chronic mental and physical illness. The level of health achieved by such groups as migrants, the poor, young children, women, the unemployed, the elderly and the chronically ill is often substantially lower than in middle class urban nuclear families (Cuthbert 1989). In all countries indigenous people are at risk for ill health. Choo (1990) reports that for Australian Aborigines 'the average life-expectancy at birth is 20 years less than for other Australians. Infant mortality is nearly three times that of non-Aboriginal children. Thirty-two percent of Aboriginal children aged 0-9 years, as against 1.6% of non-Aboriginal children, have some form of trachoma' (p. 1). Leeder and Grossman (1991) report that as we see consistent and continuing improvements in the health of the affluent, 'there is a disappointing stasis in Aboriginal health; social class gradients persist, and some health problems, such as smoking, are actually increasing' (p. 2).

To achieve equity in health care services requires more than a philosophical commitment. It requires an awareness that inequities exist in all communities, and practice strategies which demonstrate respect for and sensitivity towards vulnerable groups and individuals in the community. In many cases, the inequities are the result of a lack of access to either health care or information.

Access

As the voice of nurses world wide, the ICN has expressed its concern with the fact that over half of the 463 million married women in developing countries (excluding China) have little or no access to effective methods of birth control (ICN 1990). This has a direct effect on our greatest environmental problem: over-population. In the developed countries, access to health care is prohibited by cost-ineffective technologies and ignorance of the channels of entry. The other important factor contributing to inaccessiblity of health care is isolation, a situation about which we can do very little, and isolating attitudes, a situation which can be overcome by developing a global orientation to community health nursing and a commitment to community self-empowerment.

Empowerment

The term 'community empowerment' has become firmly embedded in the rhetoric of health for all. When two or more people share their reality they become a community which is empowered to act more effectively (Labonte 1989). Empowerment is defined by Gibson (1991) as 'a social process of recognizing, promoting and enhancing people's abilities to meet their own needs, solve their own problems and mobilize the necessary resources in order to feel in control of their own lives' (p. 359). Poverty is one of the most important issues in empowerment because the poor have a lack of control over critical resources needed to function effectively in society (Moccia & Mason 1986). Wallerstein (1992, p. 198) suggests that empowerment includes 'increased individual and community control, political efficacy, improved quality of community life, and social justice'.

Empowered communities have provided us with such popular movements as the women's movement, the environmental movement, and the occupational health movement. These movements, in turn, have informed us about diethylstilboestrol (DES), Agent Orange and other pesticides, unnecessary hysterectomies and radical mastectomies, the side effects of breast implants and asbestosis. In effect, these communities of consumers have come to recognize alienation and powerlessness as health hazards and have thus defined health according to their cultural, social and political priorities. As nurses, our role is to work in partnership with such communities, to learn from them and with them and to keep ourselves informed so that we can help them make informed choices.

Cultural sensitivity

The concept of culture is usually used to describe ethnicity or ethnic differences. However, culture has a wider meaning in society when one considers the enculturating experience of belonging to one or more groups. For example, there is a 'culture' of women, defined with increasing clarity in feminist literature. Writers such as Ann Oakley (1980), Germaine Greer (1984) and Dale Spender (1982) have identified various difficulties faced by women as a group including oppression by male-dominated societies and lack of employment opportunities related to child rearing obligations. Identification with other cultural groups also has its problems. For example, there is a culture of poverty, a drug culture and a variety of adolescent cultures. Cultural sensitivity requires that, in assessing the needs of individuals and families in the community, consideration will be given to factors related not only to the ethnic identity, but to those factors related to group identification.

Self-determinism

Of the five major principles of primary health care, self-determinism has been the most difficult to achieve. As nurses, we attempt to strike a balance between intervening in a community and allowing the community to identify its needs and select alternatives for health and health care. To encourage community self-determinism a community development approach seems to work best.

Community development is about social change. It is not merely community involvement or participation, but it is a commitment to promote self-reliance among members of a community in terms of personal and social group capacities (Dixon 1989). In other words, it is an empowering process, but one which does not blame the victim, foster illusions or confuse the issue of power. Dixon (1989) suggests that communities cannot be self-determined if they do not have power over information, relationships, decision making and resources. When health care or services are 'provided' there is a provider-consumer relationship established which often disempowers the consumer. The primary health care approach considers that the health care professional does not provide, but creates opportunities for consensus building, for relaxed communication, for sharing experiences, for developing trust (Dixon 1989). By adopting a community development approach, the nurse (or other health care worker) becomes accountable to the community, shifting the relationship to one of partnership and collaboration in choosing options for health. Community health nursing within the primary health care philosophy thus becomes primarily focused on advocacy for self-determined, community self-empowered health care.

PRIMARY HEALTH CARE AS ORGANIZATIONAL STRATEGY

One of the difficulties of achieving health for all through primary health care has been the fact that the interpretation of 'health' in the context of primary health care is not uniform. Copplestone (1991) reports that to some it has meant a basic medical service, while for others it connotes the inclusion of varying proportions of positive health services. However, the organization of primary health care requires a global approach in order to provide access to essential health care which is affordable, continuing and available where people live and work. This was the goal of representatives of the 38 nations who met in Ottawa, Canada, in 1986 to evaluate progress in achieving health for all by the year 2000 (the objective of the Declaration of Alma Ata). The Ottawa meeting produced a blueprint for the future which was called the Ottawa Charter for Health Promotion (see Fig. 1.2). The charter identified fundamental conditions and resources for health as including peace, shelter, education, food, income, a stable ecosystem, sustainable resources, social justice and equity. In order to help people achieve these conditions and resources, health professionals were urged to adopt an enabling approach, to advocate for health and to accept a major responsibility to mediate between

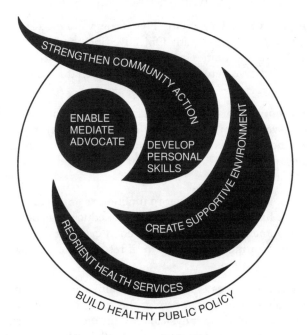

Fig. 1.2   The Ottawa Charter for Health Promotion (WHO-Health and Welfare Canada-CPHA 1986).

differing interests in society for the pursuit of health (WHO-Health & Welfare Canada-CPHA 1986). Participants at the Second International Conference on Health Promotion held in Adelaide in 1988 readily adopted this mandate as a guide to health promotion activities in Australia (Baum, Traynor & Brice 1992).

The Ottawa Charter has subsequently been dubbed the 'New Public Health' movement (Egger et al 1990). The charter's grass-roots, bottom-up approach presents a sharp contrast to the traditional organization of public health which was very much a top-down, government-prescribed system of determining health care needs. The new public health involves health promotion and disease control as well as health sector involvement in public policy planning (Egger et al 1990). In Australia, the National Better Health Program, an incentive of the Australian Health Ministers Conference, has advocated the Ottawa Charter as a strategy for implementing primary health care on a national level (National Centre for Epidemiology and Population Health/National Better Health Program 1991).

As the charter illustrates, five major strategies were proposed for health promotion. These are as follows:

Build healthy public policy. The objective of this strategy is to put health on the agenda of policy makers in all sectors and at all levels. This requires collaboration between all sectors, for example, those planning policies for health, education, manufacturing, taxation and the environment.

Create supportive environment. This strategy is aimed at encouraging a socioecological approach to health. Objectives include developing programs organized to help communities to be socially supportive of one another while attempting to conserve natural resources which enable people to maintain health.

Strengthen community action. This strategy involves adopting a community development approach to empower communities to achieve their self-defined goals. It requires access to information and learning opportunities as the basis for informed choice and most importantly, funding support.

Develop personal skills. In order to function as an enabler of health and health care, we have an obligation to provide education and opportunities for skills development. This can be achieved by capitalizing on the resources of educational institutions as well as local resources and knowledge which can be shared with others.

Reorient health services. Those in the health sector must move beyond curative and clinical services, opening the channels between health and social, political, economic physical environments. Important to this reorientation is the need for research at all levels of health care and continuing professional education for primary health care.

THE ROLE OF THE COMMUNITY HEALTH NURSE

Community health nursing practice is guided by the tenets of primary health care. In any community the nurse must assess and plan for care and caring which is equitable, accessible, culturally sensitive and which empowers the community, family or individual for self-determined health care. This may appear to be a formidable task, however, small gains at the community level are the key to achieving global goals.

The goals of primary health care are not unique to community health nursing. Primary health care is important even in the seemingly incongruous high-tech setting of the hospital. For example, when nurses in hospital provide referral to support groups, aids to facilitate daily living and developmental screening, they are engaging in primary health care (Berland 1992). Nurses in both community and institutional settings must adopt the philosophy and holistic view of health and health care. However, there are several ways in which the role of the nurse in the community differs from that of the institutionally employed nurse.

COMMUNITY HEALTH NURSING
COMPARED TO INSTITUTIONAL NURSING

The *focus* of community health nursing is primarily promotion of health and prevention of illness, rather than treatment of illness. Because of this emphasis on maintaining health and wellness, the client population do not usually define themselves as ill. In the institutional environment, nursing care revolves around the illness episode; in the community, the nurse-client relationship is continuing, rather than episodic.

The *boundaries* of the community health nursing role are much less distinct than those of the institutional nurse. The community role embodies a broad, variable range of activities, demanding a generalist, rather than specialist, orientation. As the client may include the individual, family and often the sociocultural group, the sphere of intimacy in community health nursing is broader than in the institutional environment. Community practice therefore requires a great deal of effort to be directed toward co-ordination activities. Many institutions and agencies are dealt with, and the scope of professional disciplines is wider than that encountered in the hospital setting.

An additional difference between community health and institutional nursing concerns *legal issues*. In the community, legal issues are more diverse, encompassing health related laws of particular jurisdictions as well as the relevant nurse practice Acts. The community health nurse also functions in many cases as a relatively autonomous practitioner without the legal protection of protocols, and, occasionally, without appropriate policies. This is not to imply that there is a lack of proactive planning in the community, but rather to emphasize the unpredictability of community health nursing practice (Helvie et al 1968).

Despite the unpredictability, community health nursing is guided by practice standards which define the desired and achievable range of nursing activities with which actual practice activities can be compared. Appendix 1 delineates the standards for community health nursing practice in Australia. These were developed by the Australian Council of Community Nursing Services (ACCNS) and derived from both the standards for nursing practice (published by the Australian Nursing Federation) and the standards for community nursing practice (published by the South Australian Health Commission). These standards relate to professional, communication and organizational aspects of the nursing role. The standards and their correspondent practice behaviours reflect a highly diversified role, but one which can be categorized into six general domains of community health nursing practice (Table 1.1).

Table 1.1   Domains of community health nursing practice

Management of patient health/illness in ambulatory care settings
Monitoring and ensuring the quality of health care practices
Organizational and work role competencies
The helping role
The teaching-coaching function
The consulting role

These domains are an adaptation of the list of practice domains developed by Benner (1984) in her study of clinical nurses and subsequently modified by Fenton (1985) and Brykczynski (1989) in their studies of advanced clinicians and nurse practitioners respectively. The list was validated in an analysis of the practice activities of expert nurses practising in child health, school health and district nursing in Perth, Western Australia (McMurray 1991). All nurses who participated in the study demonstrated multiple examples of domain-specific characteristics in the context of self-management and client management. Further discussion of these activities is presented in Chapter 4.

To practise within these domains, the community health nurse must have a comprehensive knowledge base and highly refined problem solving, decision making skills. He or she must have a knowledge of public health, the humanities, the social and behavioural sciences, epidemiology and nursing sciences (American Nurses Association 1986). Each of these subject areas forms an essential component which enables the nurse to participate in community development, to judge an individual's capacity for self-care and self-monitoring, and to understand individual functioning, family dynamics, patterns of human response in the face of illness and disruption, and how emotional states serve to either inhibit or potentiate health.

Community health nurses practise in a variety of settings. Some function as independent or collaborating practitioners in remote areas or urban settings such as public health, community clinics, home visiting agencies, shop front health centres and occupational health settings. Regardless of the setting, in most cases, the role is delineated in terms of the health care system and the expectations of the client population. In many health care systems nursing services are organized around specialty areas such as school health or child health while in others the nurse practises as a generalist, responsive to the needs of the community in a role which is largely that of care co-ordinator and consultant. These variations in roles and specialty areas are discussed in the chapter to follow.

SUMMARY

Community health nursing practice requires a working knowledge of health and illness, the community and its residents, and the organization and distribution of health care services. The nurse co-ordinates care to individuals, families and communities, consulting with clients and assisting them in making informed choices for health which are equitable, accessible, culturally appropriate, and practical. Although there is great diversity in the settings in which they practise, all community health nurses share one powerful unifying collegial value: respect for others, and one major goal: the health of the community. From these flow the philosophical tenets of practice: caring, nurturing and advocacy for self-empowerment. To nurse the community is to adopt the pivotal position in mobilizing communities towards health for all. To do so holistically and comprehensively is to facilitate and enable primary health care.

Study exercises

1. Provide a critique of the author's definition of health. Is it broad enough to encompass all aspects of health? What are its limitations?
2. How does the ecological model of health differ from a medical model of health?
3. Discuss five ways in which community health nurses can promote the health of a community.
4. You have been assigned to a community which is:
   a. somewhat isolated and has the following problems:
      (i) a minority group of Asian migrants who have thus far been hesitant to mix with the 'locals'
      (ii) a high incidence of childhood asthma
      (iii) a low attendance rate at the community clinic
      (iv) a lack of recreational facilities.
   b. suburban and has the following problems:
      (i) low socioeconomic status due to high unemployment
      (ii) alcoholism among the young of both sexes

(iii) both Aboriginal and non-Aboriginal residents

(iv) a high rate of single adolescent pregnancy.

c. a farming community and has the following problems:

(i) a high rate of marriage breakdowns

(ii) alcohol-related problems among the adults

(iii) a cluster of leukaemia cases

(iv) a high incidence of asthma.

How would you use the philosophy of primary health care and the strategies of the Ottawa Charter for Health Promotion to help the community?

REFERENCES

American Nurses Association, Council of Community Health Nurses 1986 ANA, Kansas City

Australian Nursing Federation 1990 Primary health care in Australia: strategies for nursing action. ANF, Melbourne

Baum F, Traynor M, Brice G 1992 Healthy cities: the Noarlunga experience. In: Gardner H (ed) Health policy development, implementation and evaluation in Australia. Churchill Livingstone, Melbourne, pp 337-360

Benner P 1984 From novice to expert: excellence and power in clinical nursing practice. Addison-Wesley, Menlo Park

Berland A 1992 Primary health care: what does it mean for nurses? International Nursing Review 39(2):42-52

Brykczynski K 1989 An interpretive study describing the clinical judgment of nurse practitioners. Scholarly Inquiry for Nursing Practice 3(2):75-104

Buttimer A 1976 Grasping the dynamism of lifeworld. Annals of the Association of American Geographers 66(2):277-292

Campbell J 1989 Place as social and geographical. In: Black D, Kunze D, Pickles J (eds) Commonplaces: essays on the nature of place. University Press of America, Lanham, Md., pp 67-79

Chamberlain M, Beckingham A 1987 Primary health care in Canada: in praise of the nurse. International Nursing Review 34(6):158-160

Choo C 1990 Aboriginal child poverty. Brotherhood of St Laurence, Melbourne

Clark M 1984 Community nursing: health care for today and tomorrow. Reston Publishing, Reston

Copplestone J 1991 What is health? World Health Forum 12(4):440-442

Cuthbert M 1989 Health maintenance organizations, primary care, and health for all by the year 2000: a critical issue for nursing. In: Gray G, Pratt R (eds) Issues in Australian nursing 2. Churchill Livingstone, Melbourne, pp 99-114

Dixon J 1989 The limits and potential of community development. Community Health Studies XIII(1):82-92

Egger G, Spark R, Lawson J 1990 Health promotion strategies & methods. McGraw-Hill, Sydney

Eng E, Salmon M, Mullan F 1992 Community empowerment: the critical base for primary health care. Family Community Health 15(1):1-12

Fenton M 1985 Identifying competencies of clinical nurse specialists. Journal of Nursing Administration 15(2):31-37

Gibson C 1991 A concept analysis of empowerment. Journal of Advanced Nursing 16:354-361

Goeppinger J, Lassiter P, Wilcox B 1982 Community health is community competence. Nursing Outlook 30:464-467

Greer G 1984 Sex and destiny: the politics of human fertility. Secker & Warburg, London

Helvie C, Hill A, Bambino C 1968 The setting and nursing practice. Nursing Outlook 16(7):27-29

Holzemer W 1992 Linking primary health care and self-care through case management. International Nursing Review 39(3):83-89

Hudson-Rodd N 1991 Place and health in Canada: historical roots of two healing traditions. Doctoral Dissertation, University of Ottawa School of Graduate Studies and Research, Ottawa

ICN-WHO 1979 The role of nursing in primary health care, report of a workshop, Nairobi, Kenya. WHO, Geneva

ICN 1990 Nurses and the environment. Geneva pp 7-9

Labonte R 1989 Community empowerment: the need for political analysis. Canadian Journal of Public Health 80(3):87-88

Lawler J 1983 Ousting Maslow from nursing. The Australian Nurses Journal 13(1): 36-38

Lawler J 1991 In search of an Australian identity. In: Gray G, Pratt R (eds) Towards a discipline of nursing. Churchill Livingstone, Melbourne, pp 211-227

Leeder S, Grossman J 1991 A din of inequity. Australian Journal of Public Health 15(1):2-4

Little C 1992 HFA by the year 2000: where is it now? Nursing & Health Care 13(4):198-201

Maglacas A 1988 Health for all: nursing's role. Nursing Outlook 36(2): 66-71

Mahler H 1979 What is health for all? World Health Nov: 3-5

Maslow A 1943 A theory of human motivation. Psychological Review 50:370-396

McDonald P 1990 Bird's-eye-view of Australia's children. Family Matters 17:7

McMurray A 1991 Expertise in community health nursing. Unpublished doctoral thesis, Department of Education, The University of Western Australia, Perth

Moccia P, Mason D 1986 Poverty trends: implications for nursing. Nursing Outlook 34(1):20

Morrow H 1988 Nurses, nursing and women. International Nursing Review 35(1):22-25

National Centre for Epidemiology and Population Health/National Better Health Program 1991 The role of primary health care in health promotion in Australia. Australian Government Publishing Service, Canberra

Nightingale F 1859 Notes on nursing: what it is and what it is not. Harrison, London

Oakley A 1980 Women confined: towards a sociology of childbirth. Martin Robertson, Oxford

Pender N 1987 Health promotion in nursing practice, 2nd edn. Appleton & Lange, Norwalk

Salmon M, Talashek M, Tichy A 1988 Health for all: a transnational model for nursing. International Nursing Review 35(4):107-109

Shotter J 1985 Accounting for place and space. Environment and Planning Vol D: Society and Space 3:447-460

Smith R, Forchuk C, Martin M 1985 Primary what? International Nursing Review 32(6):174-175, 180

Spender D 1982 Man made language. Routledge & Kegan Paul, London

Wallerstein N 1992 Powerlessness, empowerment, and health: implications for health promotion programs. American Journal of Health Promotion 6(3):197-205

Williams C 1986 Community health nursing—what is it? In: Spradley B (ed) Readings in community health nursing, 3rd edn. Little Brown, Boston, pp 67-73

WHO 1974 Basic documents 36th edn. WHO, Geneva

WHO-UNICEF 1978 Primary health care. WHO, Geneva

WHO-Health and Welfare Canada-CPHA 1986 Ottawa Charter for Health Promotion. Canadian Journal of Public Health 77(12):425-430

WHO 1989 Report on the first European conference on the environment and health. Geneva

WHO Commission on Health and Environment 1992 Health and the environment: a global challenge. Bulletin of the World Health Organization 70(4):409-413

2. Community health nursing specialties

SPECIALIZATION

Specialization in nursing has been the focus of debate for the past two decades. Bajnok (1988) explains that the generalist/specialist dichotomy was born because of the differing aims of educators and employers. From the educators' perspective, a nurse who has completed a university degree is, by virtue of the education, a generalist. Some of these graduates are employed in specialist areas, but are not considered specialists until having attained postgraduate specialist education. Employers, on the other hand, often consider experience as the determinant of specialist status. For example, in many places, the designation 'occupational health nurse' is used to denote a nurse with prior experience rather than specialist credentials in occupational health nursing. Having gained access to a specialty field through employment, the nurse typically attempts to build upon generalist knowledge, developing the competencies unique to that specialty. This represents a 'de facto' specialization which, although it may satisfy employer requirements, goes without formal recognition. Because such a small proportion of these informal specialists have the opportunity to contribute to curriculum development for other nurses, the specialty areas within community health nursing have been slow to be defined and developed. Perhaps this can be overcome if, as Benner (1984) suggests, we encourage the validation and transmission of knowledge gained through experience to successive generations of nurses.

THE SPECIALIST COMMUNITY HEALTH NURSE

The practice of community health nursing is as diverse as the clients and settings it serves. Some nurses provide health care for specific population aggregates, such as infants and children, while others provide care for all within a designated setting (for example, occupational groups). Some, by virtue of the setting, provide care for only those members of a particular aggregate who are also confined to a defined setting. The school health nurse in a secondary, or high school is an example of this. Her or his client population consists of adolescents who also share a common setting, the school. All of these nurses practise from the broad generalist knowledge base which typifies community health nursing. However, in order to meet the needs of special client populations and communities, this knowledge base must be enriched with the appropriate specialized knowledge and skills.

Community health nursing specialty areas can be arbitrarily categorized into developmental specialties, such as child health and gerontological health nursing; or situational specialties, such as occupational health or remote area nursing. However, these are somewhat artificial categorizations, as in reality the boundaries between each become obscured by practice. For example, the remote area nurse practises child health, gerontological health, school health and occupational health nursing. Regardless, as Baumgart (1988), proposes, it must be nurses who define nursing, not the setting. Community health nurses define nursing practice according to the concepts, values and commitment to primary health care. In doing so, their specialized practice is built on a unified conceptual foundation.

DEVELOPING A SPECIALIZED ROLE

In a succinct discussion of the role of the school health nurse, Oda (1985) provides some guidance for developing any specialized nursing role. She suggests that firstly, the role purpose and function must be clearly identified for oneself and others. Secondly, the role must be implemented through goal-directed interactions, and thirdly, the nurse must work toward achieving positive recognition and support for the role. She then elaborates how each of these activities is operationalized.

Role identification

The purpose and parameters of practice must be clarified and articulated based on a philosophy of practice. As Oda (1985) suggests, 'Nurses may have to gain entry to a system, negotiate their role, know *what* they will do as well as what they will *not* do, *why* they will do it, and *when* they will expect to achieve their goals to a certain degree' (p. 376). This is accomplished by prioritizing activities and articulating role limits so that the service is manageable, visible and indispensable.

Role transition

Oda (1985) suggests that an important goal for nurses in any setting is to achieve a 'role fit' by negotiating mutually acceptable expectations of what the nurse should be involved in. This requires a creative approach to communicating with others within the work setting and being flexible and responsive to the goals of others. Parsons and Felton (1992) maintain that a continuing redefinition and realignment of the role is essential for reducing ambiguity and enhancing nurses' role performance.

Role confirmation

Being accepted and respected as a professional in the work place typically proceeds through the stages of endorsement (positive ackowledgement), support, mutuality (mutual dependence), trust and autonomy (Oda 1985). The nurse's role in gaining this type of recognition lies in integrating nursing activities with other work place activities, becoming part of the referral and consulting network, and maintaining personal accountability (Oda 1985).

Regardless of specialty, community health nurses have much in common. As mentioned previously, the philosophy of primary health care provides a common conceptual foundation. Respect for the client and the right to self-determined care is paramount. Practice within all specialties is scientifically derived and regardless of whether the client enters the system through self-referral or case finding, such as occurs when there is an illness in the family, nursing activities are directed toward primary, secondary and tertiary levels of prevention.

Nursing in the community is part of a team effort, particularly when the entire community is the client and primary health care is the goal. The major advantage of a teamwork approach is that the quality of a team's vision and decision making may differ considerably from the vision of any individual's discipline or service orientation (Schofield 1992). For example, a medically dominated service may tend to equate health promotion with medical intervention, whereas the nursing perspective can help to focus on methods for behaviour change and community empowerment. Within the team and within the community the process of exploring, implementing and communicating the nursing role to others presents a common challenge. Besides these commonalities, each specialty has its own unique goals and conventions which are often not clearly understood by other nurses. The following discussion therefore provides a glimpse through the window of community health nursing at the realities of specialized practice.

Practice within each specialized area is described under the categories of primary, secondary and tertiary prevention. However, it is important to recognize that in reality, there is overlap between categories. For example, screening for hypertension in an occupational health setting may be part of the nurse's health promotion initiative, and thus may be considered primary prevention. On the other hand, in a group of workers known to have a relatively high incidence of hypertension, screening may be considered a secondary prevention activity. In addition, the three different types of activities (primary, secondary, tertiary) do not usually follow a sequential order. Most nurses move between primary, secondary and tertiary prevention activities in response to both community goals and the situation.

CHILD HEALTH NURSING

The role of the child health nurse is primarily to support and assist parents in maintaining the health of their children. In Australia the role and function of the child health nurse has historically been separate from that of other community health nurses, however, with the recent economic rationalization of health care services, some child health nursing functions are now being integrated with those of generalist community health nurses.

Child health nurses provide clinics for infants and children as well as undertaking home visits. In most cases, a clinic visit revolves around developmental assessments of children at predetermined intervals; in other cases, an 'open' clinic is conducted for parents who may wish to see the nurse regarding an unanticipated problem or issue. Developmental screening is aimed at detecting physical problems, vision, hearing or language difficulties and ascertaining whether the child is growing and developing in accordance with the normal or expected pattern. An initial developmental assessment is conducted by the nurse in the family home within the first few weeks of a child's life. These home visits are arranged with all new parents following notification of birth from the discharging hospital.

Regardless of whether the encounter is in the clinic or the home, a large proportion of the child health nurse's role involves providing advice and reassurance to the parent(s) on child care, child behaviour, feeding and nutrition. In many cases the child health nurse functions as a family nurse, practising holistically and providing parenting support. For example, some nurses run parenting education sessions, 'meet-a-parent' groups for young parents and their preschool children. Others become very involved with families as their life-line to resources and support services. Case 2.1, an excerpt from a child health nurse-client encounter illustrates this family orientation.

Case 2.1: A child health encounter

Nurse: How are you and the baby?

Mother: I have a sore nipple.

The nurse examines her nipple.

Nurse: Is it worse in certain feeding positions?

Mother: It's not *so* bad. But it makes feeding slow and I don't have time for Fred [husband] as it is.

Nurse: You're concerned about him?

Mother: He's depressed.

Nurse: Depressed?

Mother: He thinks I'm neglecting him.

At this point the mother confided her concern to the nurse that the marriage may not survive the strain of the new baby. The nurse sat and listened while the mother explained that, in addition to the birth of her child, she had also made some recent personal development choices which had proved threatening to her husband. He was reacting by exhibiting what the mother described as childish behaviour, placing undue demands on her for meals on time and accusing her of not meeting his needs. The nurse then asked the mother for her opinion on the kind of help she needed, discussed the options with her, gave her some suggestions for unblocking her nipple (which she described at this point as a relatively minor problem) and made a telephone referral to a marriage counsellor (McMurray 1991, p. 120).

According to the nurse who was being observed and interviewed in this encounter, this is fairly typical of the interaction between the child health nurse and a new mother. The clinic visit provides the opportunity to examine the child, assess whether the mother (or father) requires any assistance or parenting resources, gain an understanding of the family environment and determine the family's needs for primary, secondary and tertiary prevention activities.

Primary prevention

Primary prevention in child and family health revolves around promoting and enhancing the family's growth potential by providing anticipatory guidance. According to Bradshaw (1988) this requires a knowledge of the family's concept of health and illness, health beliefs and values, health behaviours and utilization of health services. This information is gained through the family assessment process (see Chapter 4). Anticipatory guidance usually takes the form of health teaching. The nurse may provide an overview of issues related to parenting and changing family dynamics in the course of conducting parenting classes. In addition (or alternatively), teaching sessions may be arranged on a one-to-one basis and may be appropriately timed to coincide with the child's developmental assessments. In most cases, teaching revolves around the child's physical, psychological and social development. For the family with a new baby, teaching may be aimed at providing guidance on nutrition and feeding practices (for example, when to introduce solids), immunization, teething, development of motor skills, crying patterns and other infant behaviours, and issues related to infant management such as dealing with heat, cold and nappie changes. Issues related to the family itself may include family planning and the spacing of children, the family's adjustment to a new member, dealing with the extended family, using the health care system and securing temporary respite from parenting responsibilities. For the family with a toddler, parent teaching may include any or all of the topics relevant to infants as well as discipline, sibling relationships, accident prevention, clothing, play and babysitters. The family with a school-aged child will also require information on cognitive skills development and psychosocial patterns (Dickenson-Hazard 1992).

In addition to health teaching, the nurse may also engage in primary prevention by role modelling during the course of clinic or home visits. Behaviours such as talking to the infant or child, cuddling and safe handling during dressing, undressing or feeding may provide examples for parents who would not think to ask whether to chat to their child, how to hold their infant securely, or how to communicate love and affection to the child whenever he or she is being handled.

Secondary prevention

For the child health nurse secondary prevention activities usually arise in response to a parental request for help or information. For example, many nurses act as an interpreter of the health care system. Parents who have visited their family physician or specialist often rely on the nurse to explain what he or she meant by 'don't feed so often', 'watch the baby's stools', 'give the child lots of fluids', 'keep an eye on the swelling' and other rather vague instructions which leave the parents in a quandary about the meaning of such terms as 'often' and 'lots'.

Secondary prevention also includes instructing parents on special care needs and treatments for the infant or child with acute or chronic illness or who has been injured, counselling parents whose child has been the victim of trauma or a congenital abnormality and teaching them how to deal with childhood diseases, chronic illnesses and/or hospitalization. Once difficulties have been identified the nurse may also provide family counselling or referral to local resources which provide support services.

Tertiary prevention

Nursing actions which help parents through the process of rehabilitation or health maintenance following illness or injury constitute tertiary prevention. This may include ongoing support for the family, liaison with other members of the health care team and self-help groups, as well as long term counselling while families adjust to changing circumstances or lifestyles. Usually tertiary prevention requires home visits to provide realistic guidance for the family which is within their economic and social capability. For example, to suggest that a young mother secure a babysitter and go out shopping to enhance her self-esteem may be totally inappropriate for the family living below the poverty line. Similarly, to suggest that a husband, rather than an older sister take care of the children while a mother attended an appointment may, in an Aboriginal family, be culturally inappropriate. The child health nurse who is able to maintain an ongoing relationship with a family during its child bearing years has a special primary health care responsibility, for she or he has an opportunity to facilitate some of the family's most important functions:

child rearing, evolving with the various stages of family development and achieving and maintaining culturally congruent health.

COMMUNITY MENTAL HEALTH NURSING

Mental health is defined by Clark (1984) as 'a dynamic state in which equilibrium is maintained by a precarious balance between stressors and resources' (p. 447). It is a function of the cumulative impact of many variables. Psychologically healthy behaviour is related to age, developmental stage, family and social support systems, cultural mores, the environment and the activities of others. Other factors influencing mental health include the rate and number of changes occurring in a given time in a person's life and whether or not these are viewed as disruptive to psychological equilibrium; and the individual's coping ability (Lancaster & Kerschner 1988). Optimal mental health is a state in which the individual feels self-worth and self-fulfilment, enjoys comfortable relationships with others and has a sense of mastery over the environment (Clark 1984).

Facilitating and enabling mental health is integral to the delivery of holistic health care as mental and physical health are inextricably entwined. Physical health or illness can be precipitated, intensified or enhanced by psychological states. Psychological states are reciprocally affected by physical states. Both are affected by cultural and societal factors. It is a familiar axiom that this era which has provided technological conquests over many illnesses has produced a corresponding number of stressors. Current threats to mental health include increased violence against people and property, substance abuse, family breakdowns, inflation, unemployment and the difficulties for women of having to maintain the dual roles of worker and family caretaker (Lancaster & Kerschner 1988). To this list one could add the pervasive threat of nuclear accidents or nuclear war, environmental pollution and crowding, information overload, the difficulties of guiding children through the confused morality and values of contemporary society and the distorted images of life created by the media in the name of entertainment. All of these issues have a profound effect on the health of a community and therefore are the concern of the community health nurse.

Epidemiological data reveal that there is a significant level of psychological morbidity in the community. The Australian Health Ministers estimate that 1 in 5 Australians will, at some point in their lives, experience significant disruption to their mental well being and quality of life (Commonwealth of Australia 1992). For most mental disorders, women show higher levels than men, particularly for depression, anxiety states and somatization disorders (NH&MRC 1991). Contrary to the myths surrounding the influence of female hormones in mental states, Jorm (1987) found that peaks and rises in the morbidity data related to depression do not fit with hormonal patterns. Rather, he suggests, mental states are related to social role differentiation and social circumstances such as low socioeconomic status and lack of social support networks. These are important factors when considering the 'feminization of poverty' which occurs with many separated mothers, elderly single females with no means of financial support and many migrant women. The report of the Health Care Committee Expert Advisory Panel on Women and Mental Health (NH&MRC 1991) suggests that the mental health of women must be viewed in the context of the impact of structural issues in society which include not only poverty, but power, competing roles, socialization and bias in some health professionals. These factors not only constitute stressors for women, but 'in many cases influence their presentations, their behaviour, interpretations, distress and needs' (NH&MRC 1991, p. 7).

The National Mental Health Policy advances the position that a community-oriented approach to the provision of mental health services has demanded a new relationship between mental health services and the wider health sector in order to move these services closer to family, community and cultural networks (Commonwealth of Australia 1992). To function as advocate for a community's mental health, therefore, requires the holistic, population-focused approach of primary health care. As a primary health care provider, the community mental health nurse functions as a co-ordinator of primary, secondary and tertiary prevention activities, and often as a consultant to other health care providers.

Primary prevention

Primary prevention in mental health nursing involves the promotion of adaptive strengths and coping resources. This takes the form of public education and consultation on mental health issues, and preventive activities which focus on those at risk for mental ill health. Groups who are at risk for psychological problems include women; young people; those in the lowest social classes; the elderly; migrants and others experiencing social isolation; families undergoing separation and/or with chronically ill or handicapped members and victims of aggression or crime (Clark 1984, Porter 1985). Community health nurses can contribute to helping these vulnerable groups by participating in professional and interdisciplinary groups aimed at heightening awareness of mental health issues by engaging in political lobbying for improved social conditions, and by conducting health education programs for individuals, groups and communities.

Health education program must focus on high risk situations (giving birth in a new culture, coping with crisis in the family) as well as high risk groups (migrants, young mothers). Special programs may be designed around such topics as parenting, stress management, assertiveness, smoking, substance abuse, self-health and retirement (Berns & Hamilton 1985, Porter 1985, Lancaster & Kerschner 1988). Nurses can also contribute to the mental health needs of the community by participating in programs and public awareness campaigns which attempt to overcome the societal problems of marital breakdown, environmental pollution, unemployment, homelessness, isolation, discrimination, and political subjugation, all of which compromise a community's quality of life. In many cases, this involves liaison with other sectors of society. For example, in order to promote the health and well being of homeless youth, Burdekin et al (1989) recommended a collaborative approach between the health, legal, education, housing and employment sectors.

Natural support systems such as friends, neighbours and indigenous helpers (for example, Aboriginal health workers) can also be invaluable intermediaries for health education. Community groups comprise an important component of the community resource network as well as providing support and reinforcement for health promotion. Furthermore, the nurse's membership in local church, women's issues or self-help groups often provides legitimization for these organizations and assists with the recruitment of new members (Clark 1984).

Secondary prevention

Secondary prevention often involves crisis intervention. Crises may be categorized as situational crises, victim crises or developmental crises. A situational crisis is one which arises from a distressing event or experience, such as losing a job, undergoing a divorce, or dealing with accidental death or property damage. A victim crisis is one in which the individual is traumatized, injured or destroyed physically or psychologically. Rape and natural disasters fall into this category. Developmental crises are those which are associated with the developmental stages of life, such as adolescence, marriage, the birth of a first child or retirement (Berns & Hamilton 1985). The object of crisis intervention is to decrease the duration or intensity of dysfunction. The nurse attempts to do this by prompt case finding and early intervention to minimize long term impairment and prevent hospitalization. This is called case management and involves two goals: to link clients with appropriate community-based services and to establish a therapeutic plan which would rationalize the provision of services to reduce inappropriate use of expensive inpatient care (Holzemer 1992). The therapeutic plan can involve any combination of physical care, education, counselling, or referral to individual or group therapy.

The most important target group for secondary prevention is the individual and the family undergoing marital breakdown or divorce. The nurse needs to assess individual situations in terms of the family itself and each member's ability to cope (see also Ch. 4). In a study of non-custodial mothers' relationships with their children following separation and divorce it was found that financial pressures and lack of social support were major factors which interfered with the mothers' ability to maintain warm and nurturing parent-child relationships (McMurray 1992). All members of separating families need acceptance and non-judgemental understanding. It is important to assess whether the children's reactions are within the normal ranges for their ages, whether they have the support of others, such as the non-custodial parent, or whether there is a need for counselling. Adjustment difficulties in the child which are often detected by school health nurses, or reported during visits to the child health clinic, may manifest themselves as tearfulness, aggressive outbursts, withdrawal, apathy, concentration and learning difficulties, excessive or repetitive behaviours or regression to an earlier stage.

Parents may also require support and guidance. Many times, the divorcing parents become so involved in their own feelings that they have limited energy and resources to share with their children (Lancaster & Kerschner 1988). The nurse can then be of assistance by acknowledging the difficulties of coping as well as helping them to identify and deal with any of the children's behaviours which signal adjustment problems.

A further target for secondary prevention relates to the distressing contemporary problem of homelessness. Many people today are without homes due to economic problems, unemployment or urban renewal schemes which have left them evicted from low cost dwellings, or, in the case of youth, because of family breakdowns (Burdekin et al 1989). Sebastian (1992) suggests that discharged psychiatric patients are particularly vulnerable to homelessness because of their limited resources and abilities, however, the research has not revealed whether psychiatric disorders are a cause or a consequence of homelessness (Winkleby et al 1992).

In planning nursing care for the homeless, there is little that can be done immediately for the sleep deprivation and hypothermia which plague the homeless. Nevertheless, the nurse can sometimes organize refuge, clothes and food, and provide physical care for foot problems, lacerations, infections or chronic illnesses. The nurse's major contribution to helping the homeless involves participating in community advocacy networks with others concerned with unemployment, poverty, housing and safety. This includes liaising and consulting with welfare agencies, the police and legal aid departments, firefighters, religious and other non-governmental agencies, and other care givers in order to promote co-ordination of care giving efforts.

Tertiary prevention

Tertiary prevention is aimed at reducing the residual effects of chronic mental illness and, often, of institutionalization (Porter 1985). Education, counselling and advocacy are the predominant means by which this type of psychosocial rehabilitation is accomplished (Boyer & Heppner 1992).

In synchrony with the trend towards community-based health care, is a widespread movement to deinstitutionalize the mentally ill. This has necessitated the development of community after-care programs to assist clients with activities of daily living during the transition from institution to community, and to provide a link to community resources. After-care or continuity of care programs are usually part of the discharge plan, and include direct services, such as counselling, skills assessment, and instruction and supervision of medication regimes; provision of support and anticipatory guidance for the family; community networking and co-ordinated, flexible case management (Berns & Hamilton 1985, Lancaster & Kerschner 1988,

Boyer & Heppner 1992). According to Lancaster and Kerschner (1988), programs for the deinstitutionalized individual need to achieve a balance between ensuring as much liberty and freedom as possible, and providing structure, medical care and a social network. Often the least restrictive and most helpful alternative for the mentally ill individual is a return to the family. However, careful monitoring may be necessary to ensure that the adjustment difficulties of the family member does not diminish the quality of life for the rest of the family (Lancaster & Kerschner 1988).

These authors identify three groups who are most affected by deinstitutionalization. The first of these is the young chronically ill who do not consider themselves as patients and are particularly vulnerable to abuses of alcohol and mind altering drugs. Another group which is particularly prone to adjustment problems is the mentally ill elderly. Deinstitutionalization often displaces them from the only home they have known. Compounding their difficulties are persistent shortages of affordable housing, poverty, and frequently, a lack of family supports. The third group who encounter difficulties in adjusting to the community is the intellectually disabled. These individuals may display emotional disorders which range from transient behaviour disturbances to psychosis. This is exacerbated in retarded or mentally deficient clients who may be non-verbal or demonstrate low self-esteem, primitive defense mechanisms and diminished coping abilities, and many also have congenital disorders with allied medical needs (Lancaster & Kerschner 1988).

In order to co-ordinate care and resources in any community, the community health nurse must be cognizant of the dynamics and constituents of mental health and mental ill health, as a community's mental health status is perhaps the most accurate predictor of its ability to adapt and evolve with societal change. To neglect a community's mental health needs is therefore to jeopardize its very survival.

SCHOOL HEALTH NURSING

The major goal of school health nursing is to enable health, and ultimately learning, in the school environment. The three core components of school health are therefore health services, health education and a healthy environment (Igoe & Speer 1992). The primary focus of school health nursing is the student, however, in practice, the nurse often attends to the health needs of school staff, parents and the families of both students and staff.

School health nurses practise in a variety of circumstances. Some are employed by local health departments to provide service to one or more schools, while others are employed by a particular school division or district to attend to the needs of the schools within their jurisdiction. In some cases, the nurse is employed to care for the primary school population of a certain school division, while another is responsible for its secondary or high school. Private schools usually have a school health nurse who is responsible for all students, whether primary school or secondary school level. Many private boarding schools have a school health nurse who lives at the school and is available to the students beyond normal school hours if necessary. In addition to the employment arrangements, Withrow (1988) attributes the diversity in the school health nursing role to the following factors:

- The nurse's education
- The role the nurse is expected to play
- The program itself
- Legal and bureaucratic constraints with which school health goals are pursued
- The size of the school division or district
- Local characteristics and values
- Availability of resources
- The ability of the nurse.

Despite the diverse nature of the role, school health nurses share many similarities. Withrow (1988) identifies seven roles of the school health nurse. The first of these is a functional role which may involve screening and subsequent follow up, communicable disease control or immunization. A second role which is performed to a greater or lesser extent by most school health nurses is primary care. This can involve direct health services such as first aid, arranging screening programs or teaching health education classes. A third role is that of team co-ordinator as all school health nurses function within a team. The team may comprise a physician, school counsellor, psychologist, social worker, physical education teacher and classroom teacher. Teams may not be visible at all times, as they are problem oriented and activated when a problem arises. A fourth role of the nurse is that of nurse practitioner. In this capacity the nurse identifies students at risk for specific health problems, manages certain chronic and/or acute health concerns and provides comprehensive and continuous programs for care. The fifth primary role is that of nurse teacher, wherein the nurse attempts to teach health concepts and provide support for changes in health behaviour. The sixth and seventh roles of the school health nurse, those of consultant and advocate, are described by Withrow as secondary roles. The nurse consultant provides consultation to the physician, school counsellor, social worker, principal, teachers, parents and other nurses. As an advocate, the nurse represents the interests of individual students, special need groups, children in the school, and the community, bureaucratic and political arenas (Withrow 1988). Within the context of these roles, the practice activities of the school health nurse are directed towards primary, secondary and tertiary levels of prevention.

Primary prevention

Primary prevention in the school consists of activities designed to promote health and to protect against disease (Withrow 1988, Igoe & Speer 1992).

Health promotion programs may be focused on themes which connect the school with the broader community. For example, the nurse may be involved in special campaigns such as the 'Jump Rope For Heart' program promoted by local and national Heart Foundations during Heart Health Month. Similarly, information and poster displays may be assembled to link health promotion activities in the school to the national AIDS awareness day. Another area in which the nurse plays a pivotal health promotion role is that of nutrition awareness. Promotion of healthy eating habits may take the form of posters, classroom information sessions, and providing guidance to those running the school canteen or snack bar. A useful health promotion tool is the school newsletter, whereby the nurse can maintain a continuing dialogue with school staff, reminding them of seasonal hazards such as sunburn in summer, influenza in winter, or the availability of health services and community resources. Igoe and Speer (1992) suggest that all health education programs conducted in the school should be family-centred and therefore be related to the values and beliefs of students and their families.

Health education in the school often involves the classroom teaching of health topics, although in some schools where the health education curriculum is taught by others, the nurse serves as a consultant, occasional guest teacher or teacher resource. Health education topics are selected to be appropriate to the school population as well as the curriculum. In primary school, lessons are generally biologically oriented, focusing on teaching children how their bodies function, and how to stay healthy. Safety is also a major focus for younger children, with information being provided on hazards in and around the home, school and the environment.

School health education programs are continually being updated to respond to current social problems. Many schools now provide resources such as videotapes, films and printed materials on self-esteem, interpersonal communications, environmental hazards, child sexual abuse, divorce and custody issues, sexually transmitted diseases, substance abuse and adolescent pregnancy. Such materials are designated according to whether the target group consists of young children or adolescents, and serve as a guide for the nurse engaged in educating staff, students and occasionally, their parents. In secondary, or high schools, health education often consumes a disproportionate percentage of the nurse's day, with topics revolving around sexuality and sexually transmitted diseases, family planning, dietary issues, alcohol and drug consumption and family relationships.

In the process of maturing, many adolescents go through a period in which their energies are directed at developing an identity distinct from the family, which often results in a temporary period of alienation. During this same period, however, there is often a need for advice and information on health issues which must be provided in an atmosphere of support and acceptance. In many cases it is the nurse who is cast into this teacher-nurturer role, bridging the gap between the adolescent and the family, teachers or other authority figures.

Primary prevention activities also include creating a healthful school environment (Igoe & Speer 1992). In this respect, school health nursing resembles occupational health nursing, as the school nurse may be called upon to conduct safety and health surveillance and monitoring of hazardous substances or conditions.

Screening and immunization programs are additional areas of primary prevention in the school. Screening programs are usually developed according to state or provincial health department priorities, and may include a variety of screening programs for vision, hearing, growth and development, scoliosis or dental problems. Other screening programs may be initiated by the school health nurse; for example, screening for pediculosis.

Immunization programs are also provided according to health department standards, and are often conducted by the department's immunization nurses who rely on the school health nurse to organize the immunization clinics. In some cases, however, immunizations such as tetanus antitoxin and influenza vaccine are administered by the school health nurse.

Secondary prevention

Secondary prevention activities involve attending to emergency situations, providing direct care of ill or injured students, prompt case finding, referral to appropriate resources when necessary, counselling and follow up. The two most challenging activities for the school health nurse are case finding and counselling. Case finding involves identification of students requiring intervention for a problem or issue. There are deliberate steps which the nurse can take to identify such students. The absentee list and the health centre statistics can be checked periodically to identify those with recurring illness, or those whose frequent visits may be masking an underlying emotional problem. Incident or accident surveys can also be conducted. In addition, the nurse must encourage teachers to identify students who simply appear ill (Withrow 1988).

Counselling involves encouraging students to make positive choices for healthful living. A counsellor's responsibility is 'to provide information, to listen objectively and to be supportive, caring and trustworthy' (Withrow 1988, p. 781). These characteristics are within most nurses' communication proficiencies, however, counselling is frequently cited by school health nurses as the most contentious aspect of the role. To be an effective counsellor requires an abundance of patience, self-confidence, thoughtful reasoning, a comprehensive inventory of resources and an understanding of the transient and enduring issues confronting students.

In some cases, students refer themselves for counselling, but in other cases, a student will be referred by teachers or parents to the school guidance counsellor. Many students, however, often look for guidance from the person with whom they have established rapport and trust, and in some cases, this is the school health nurse. Occasionally, the counselling needs of the student are beyond the capabilities of the nurse, and a decision must be made as to the most appropriate person to fulfil the counsellor role. The student may ultimately be counselled by the school guidance counsellor, by the nurse with consultation from the guidance counsellor, or by a counsellor from outside the school. If counselling is provided by someone other than the nurse, the nurse attempts to maintain liaison between the student, the counsellor, the family if they are involved and occasionally, the teacher or principal.

One important counselling challenge concerns adolescent pregnancy. The pregnant teenager may seek help from the school health nurse when she first suspects pregnancy, or once she has had her pregnancy confirmed. At either stage, she needs a non-judgemental and supportive attitude. Quite often, the adolescent responds to pregnancy with a wide range of emotions. Initially these may include denial, fear, guilt, anger, depression or happiness (Dickenson-Hazard 1988). The nurse can assist her by encouraging exploration of her feelings about pregnancy, about the options available to her, her support network and her short term goals (Dickenson-Hazard 1988).

For the pregnant adolescent who continues with the pregnancy, the importance of antenatal care must be emphasized. In addition, the nurse attempts to ensure that the adolescent understands the need to make realistic preparations for the child's arrival both physically and psychologically. If the mother will be returning to school, the nurse may also attempt to assist with study and child care arrangements, or refer her to an alternative school or agency for home study. In the situation where the adolescent chooses either abortion or to give the child up for adoption, the nurse must maintain a non-judgemental attitude, respecting the adolescent's decision. At this stage, the nurse assumes the role of resource person or health consultant. As an additional intervention, the nurse may provide a referral to group counselling or an agency which provides interaction with, and peer support from other pregnant adolescents (Dickenson-Hazard 1992). At the appropriate time, the subject of family planning should be broached with the adolescent and, if possible, with her partner. This can be aided by materials provided by the local family planning association, which is often an invaluable resource to the school health nurse.

An additional issue which often involves counselling concerns interpersonal relationships. One nurse who participated in the author's study on practice expertise commented that adolescents have a constant need for reassurance in the area of interpersonal relationships. In her words: 'Sometimes it's to do with school, sometimes with the opposite sex, and relationships, like first going to the movies or to the school ball—worrying about who's going to take whom—there are so many dramas around school ball time and they all need reassuring' (McMurray 1991, p. 130).

Another school health nurse in the same study concurred, explaining the importance of understanding interpersonal relationships for both students and teachers in the school setting. She commented: 'I do a lot of listening and give an immense amount of reassurance to students and teachers.

Communication skills are absolutely vital. You have to co-operate and get the best out of people' (McMurray 1991, p. 163).

Tertiary prevention

Tertiary prevention activities include rehabilitating the student with an illness or health issue, providing for students with disabilities, and assisting students with behaviour change and decision making (Withrow 1988). Students returning to school following an acute illness episode have varying rehabilitation needs. For some, the nurse's involvement is confined to a follow up visit and recording the student's return to school. Others may require periodic monitoring to record progress following an illness, injury or medical intervention. For example, when a student returns to school in a plaster cast, the nurse usually assesses the affected area at regular intervals to provide guidance to the student and his or her family on the management of the rehabilitation regime. Ideally, communication between the school nurse and the student's physician is maintained. However, due to time constraints and the logistical difficulties of contacting a physician for every ill or injured student, the physician is usually only contacted when the situation is questionable or further medical care is required.

Within most school populations are students with disabilities which are not totally self-managed, and/or students with chronic illness, such as diabetes, cancer, arthritis, asthma or a heart condition. Depending upon the individual situation, the nurse's involvement with a student having a physical or learning disability or who is chronically ill may be intensive and sustained. In such cases, every attempt must be made to maintain open communication between the nurse, the student, his or her family, the physician, and the teacher. At times, this makes it very difficult for the school health nurse to preserve confidentiality. However, the amount and type of information made available to those other than the health team can often be decided upon within a case conference involving the student, family and team members.

Confidentiality, and indeed the management of the school health nursing service, is dependent upon accurate and appropriate documentation. Most schools have standardized student health records which document a student's general health status and history of immunizations, screening results, illnesses and/or injuries. In addition to individual records, it is helpful to compile periodic statistics on health issues being identified in the school. These statistics indicate epidemiological trends within the school, such as the occurrence of infectious diseases, patterns of injury or illness, and health education needs. This information can then be used to draw comparisons with other schools or other geographic locations, to form the basis for program planning and policy development.

One policy which has a place in all schools is that of providing for those with disabilities. Most schools are being constructed today with concessions such as wheelchair access ramps, modified toilets and desks. In some cases, however, the nurse must advocate and agitate for alterations which would accommodate those students with physical limitations.

Besides chronic illnesses and disabilities, tertiary prevention activities must also be directed at the contemporary health issues affecting children and adolescents today. Some of the problems which require rehabilitation in the school were discussed in relation to mental health nursing (i.e. substance abuse and homelessness). Other issues which emerge in school health nursing include obesity and abuse of weight control, such as anorexia and bulimia.

Obesity is a threat to health at all stages of life, but for the child it can be the trigger to developing a lifetime of low self-esteem (Blank Sherman et al 1992). The obese child therefore needs emotional support as well as help in losing weight (Berger 1983). This presents a doubly difficult challenge in that firstly, dieting in childhood may be detrimental to the child's bone and brain growth; and secondly, eating patterns are fostered by family traditions and attitudes (Berger 1983). Childhood weight control programs must therefore concentrate on increased exercise rather than decreased dietary intake, complemented by nutritional guidance for the family. One approach to the problem is to devise an intervention and maintenance program of incremental exercise and nutrition counselling as a co-operative venture between the child, the family, the physician, the school health nurse and the physical education teacher. The school health nurse can be the source of encouragement, support and guidance for the student, the teacher and the family.

Despite the advantages of overcoming obesity at an early age, weight control programs begun in early childhood must guard against encouraging excessive weight consciousness, which may contribute to dieting abuses in adolescence or pre-adolescence. Two such abuses are anorexia nervosa and bulimia. Anorexic individuals tend to restrict their food intake and exercise to the extreme, while the bulimic person consumes large intakes of food, then purges, either by vomiting or laxative abuse (Withrow 1988). Bulimia is much more common than anorexia and is often associated with alcohol abuse or depression (Beckman Blomquist 1992). In many cases, the school health nurse is unaware of the student with eating disorders, as societal norms support weight consciousness, and minor deviations are not identified through normal school screening mechanisms. Following the diagnosis of an eating disorder a long term individual or family counselling program is usually instituted, with the school health nurse providing support for the student and family throughout the duration of therapy.

Other problems which are being seen with increasing frequency in the school setting include child physical and sexual abuse. With increasing public awareness of these problems, education departments have alerted teachers to the typical signs and symptoms of the abused child (sleepiness, apathy, withdrawal, incontinence). In many cases, when a teacher suspects abuse, the child is referred to the pastoral care team in the school. The pastoral care team usually consists of the nurse, social worker, school guidance officer, a member of the teaching staff, and in some cases, a spiritual counsellor. Team members collaborate in devising a strategy for helping the student and others in the community by ensuring that the local child abuse unit is notified and arranging for ongoing counselling and support for the victim. Where no pastoral care team exists in the school, the teacher often refers the student to the nurse, who must attempt to develop a trusting relationship with the child without pressuring him or her to divulge painful details all at once, and to ensure that the appropriate agencies are notified. According to school health nurses interviewed the important thing in dealing with these children is to build the relationship at the child's own pace and to work towards confronting the problem while maintaining a network of resources for ongoing support and counselling (McMurray 1991). This is often accomplished with the help of the school psychologist and other members of the pastoral care team. Central to the nurse's role is meticulous documentation of all encounters with the child and as much assessment information (physical, psychological and social) as possible. The nurse's role in any kind of child abuse is to act as advocate for the student, liaising with resources and all those involved with nurturing the student through the transition period of rehabilitation.

OCCUPATIONAL HEALTH NURSING

The Australian Occupational Health Nurses Association (AOHNA) defines the occupational health nurse as one who is engaged in the conservation, promotion and restoration of the health of persons at their place of work. 'Their primary goal is the prevention of occupational illness and injury. The outcome is reduced economic and social costs for both employer and employees' (AOHNA 1991, p. 3).

The role of the occupational health nurse is described by AOHNA as essentially preventive, and one which may encompass the following eight functional areas of responsibility which are dependent upon the knowledge and experience of the nurse:

1. Management of the occupational health service
2. Assessment of the work environment
3. Assessment of workers' health
4. Provision of health care
5. Training and health promotion
6. Rehabilitation of ill and injured employees
7. Maintenance of records
8. Research.

(AOHNA 1991, p. 5)

Occupational health nursing extends the goals of primary health care to the work place. The nurse practises in partnership with the worker, worker groups and the employer to plan health care which is accessible, self-determined and part of a comprehensive and continuing health care process.

The uniqueness of occupational health nursing is manifest through the advocacy role. The nurse must function as advocate for both employee and employer. This bilateral advocacy is occasionally a daunting task which requires diplomacy and strong communication skills, an understanding of interpersonal and industrial relations, and familiarity with professional and government standards and legislation. Other factors which influence occupational health nursing practice include socioecological trends (such as environmental concerns), geographic location, company and union philosophy and policies, budgetary restraints and the nurse's educational opportunities, professional support and job description.

The occupational health nurse must develop skills in hazard recognition, epidemiology, program planning, research, evaluation and organizational methods (Ray 1985). All of these activities are facilitated by team participation. Depending upon the size of the company, the inhouse team may consist of any or all of the nurse, physician, toxicologist, industrial hygienist, physiotherapist, work area supervisor, plant safety manager, personnel officer, plant manager and union shop steward (Ray 1985). According to Ossler (1992), occupational health and safety problems have become increasingly complex as a result of the interactions between biopsychosocial factors in the home, work and community environments. Because the occupational environment is itself considered a community, health care is provided according to primary, secondary and tertiary levels of prevention.

Primary prevention

At the level of primary prevention, the occupational health nurse co-ordinates health promotion and health education programs, conducts health screening, assesses the patterns of work place illness and injuries, and maintains surveillance on the work environment in which they occur (Ray 1985, Ossler 1988). In consultation with management and employee groups, the nurse may also participate in the formulation and ongoing revision of company health policy. In many cases, the nurse is attached to the personnel department, and on occasion, may participate in the formulation of employee personnel policies, such as those relating to maternity leave or day care.

Occupational health and safety legislation is primarily aimed at ensuring healthy and safe working conditions, whereas work place health promotion is concerned with the individual's physical and psychological health and the effect this has both in the work place and outside it (Quinlan & Bohle 1991). Some companies acknowledge the value of work place health and fitness programs while others consider such programs unnecessary. In some cases, it is up to the nurse to 'market' health promotion programs in such a way as to argue the economic as well as health outcomes. From his Canadian research Shepherd (1986) suggests that the industrial benefit from fitness/lifestyle programs is $513/worker/year calculated on the basis of worker satisfaction, productivity, lower absenteeism, turnover, injuries and health insurance premiums. Other studies have looked at the cost benefit of helping employees to quit smoking. Kristein (1982) identifies the potential savings of a non-smoking employee as $512/worker/year on the basis of absenteeism, productivity, fire, worker's compensation and accidents. It is, however, difficult to draw comparisons between countries and between industries because of differing work cultures and differing expectancies from single target (smoking) and multilevel programs.

Since its inception in 1985, Worksafe Australia has provided occupational health nurses and others with current and relevant data from which to plan programs. Morris (1989) reports that the annual cost of work place death and injury in Australia is $10 billion. With the inclusion of compensation and other costs the annual total cost of accidents is between 3-6% of Australia's Gross National Product (NOHSC 1988). Less tangible costs include the impact that illness may have on the morale, motivation, job satisfaction and loyalty of those workers who suffer injury or witness illnesses/injuries or their ramifications (Quinlan & Bohle 1991).

Health promotion programs cover a wide range of topics. Most occupational health nurses attempt to provide programs promoting general health, such as heart health programs or, more specifically, smoking cessation, nutrition and alcohol awareness programs. AIDS presents a unique challenge in occupational health promotion in that the majority of HIV positive people are symptomless and are active participants in the work force. Because AIDS/HIV infection is not legally notifiable, moral and ethical dilemmas such as screening policies must be resolved by individual employers. Advocacy for employees thus requires educating and informing employees of safe working practices and encouraging employers to adopt anti-discriminatory practices.

Some health promotion programs target issues peculiar to the work environment. For example, in many industries, educational programs can be devised to address the effects of shiftwork, exposure to infectious diseases or back injuries. Health education programs are often conducted as a joint effort between the nurse and safety officer or safety committee. These include programs for hearing and vision conservation, programs to educate employees in first-aid and cardiopulmonary resuscitation (CPR), and programs which are aimed at persuading the worker to wear safety equipment and take safety precautions.

Health and safety programs adopt a variety of approaches, involving posters, pamphlets, seminars, information sessions or safety contests, and some include the family of the worker. For example, an information sheet or newsletter may be distributed via the employee's pay cheque containing helpful advice on such diverse issues as parenting, menopause or cancer prevention. This is a useful means of encouraging either the worker or family members to be in contact with the nurse for additional information, or to discuss other health needs or community resources.

Screening programs are an additional component of occupational health education. Health screening is usually begun at the time of the pre-employment examination. Any pertinent health problems arising at this time can be discussed with the individual worker, and a plan for follow up or health counselling instituted. Information gained from pre-employment screening provides the nurse with a demographic profile of the worker population, which can be of assistance in identifying social and cultural influences on the employee's health as well as establishing potential risk groups.

Some occupational risk groups are related to age and sex. According to Ossler (1992), males within the 18 to 30 age group who have had less than 6 months' experience in their current job run the greatest risk for occupational injury. This is attributed to undeveloped dexterity and the possibility of risk taking, or drug and alcohol abuse. Older workers may be at risk because of their diminished sensory abilities, the effects of chronic illness or their delayed reaction time. Women in their child bearing years may occasionally experience debilitating levels of premenstrual tension or dysmennorhoea. Many women also work under relatively high stress levels as a result of the dual responsibilities of work and home. Migrant workers, particularly migrant women, are a unique risk group for occupational injury, as many of them have communication problems associated with an unfamiliar language, and may misunderstand health and safety advice (Commonwealth-State Council on Non-English Speaking Background Women's Issues 1991). The occupational health nurse can often help to bridge the cultural gap for these employees by acting as an intermediary between worker and supervisor, and between worker and community resources and support groups.

The pre-employment examination also aids in identifying employees for risks unrelated to age, sex or work experience. In most occupational environments, employees are hired with illnesses or disabilities which do not impair their work functions. The existence of these conditions must be documented in case a situation arises in which the condition predisposes the employee to occupational risk. For example, the employee with epilepsy may be suited to a position in the company purchasing department, but a subsequent change of job driving heavy equipment may prove dangerous. Such individuals can be monitored by the nurse to ensure the maintenance of a functional standard of health.

In addition to pre-employment screening, specific screening programs may also be instituted by the occupational health nurse as a parallel process to screening in the general community. Some of these include blood pressure, skin cancer, respiratory and diabetes screening programs. Another growing area of nurse involvement in the work place is pre-retirement counselling, which can be conducted individually or in groups. Some companies contract to have a retirement counsellor provide programs for their employees, while others offer a team approach, with the nurse covering health care topics.

Work place surveillance and safety audits are an additional measure taken for primary prevention. Depending upon the size of the company, the nurse may be responsible for safety promotion, or may function as a member of the safety surveillance team. To be effective, the nurse must be familiar with the industry, its individual jobs, the equipment used in the conduct of various jobs, and the environment in which each job is undertaken.

Surveys must be conducted periodically to detect ergonomic, physical, psychosocial, biologic or chemical hazards (Ossler 1992). Ergonomics is the study of the engineering aspects of the relationship between human workers and their work environment, that is, the person-machine interface. Most government departments of occupational health and safety provide resources to guide ergonometric assessment, and there are many texts available on the subject. However, the most useful way to gain an understanding of each work setting is to interview the workers, supervisors and the plant manager, then to spend some time observing each job as it is being performed. As time consuming as this is, it should be standard procedure for any nurse upon first entering an occupational health position, to aid in making accurate assessments of work place hazards or injuries, and to convey a sense of understanding to the worker of his or her particular job. Ossler (1992) identifies ergonomically deficient work tasks as those which create fatigue, boredom, glare, or which must be conducted in an abnormal position. Examples are vibration, repetitive motion, poor workstation-worker fit and the lifting of heavy loads.

Physical hazards include extremes of temperature, noise radiation and lighting. Psychosocial hazards are those which produce inordinate amounts of stress, such as rotational shiftwork and negative interpersonal relationships on the job. Biologic hazards include bacteria, moulds, insects, viruses or fungi; while chemical hazards may include liquids, gases, mist, dust particulates, vapours or fumes (Ossler 1992).

The hazard survey, combined with illness and injury statistics, contributes to the database of work place risk. These data, together with the information obtained through screening, provide the nurse with a basis to consult with management on the development of programs for risk management and promotion of optimal work place health and safety.

A final activity for primary prevention, concerns the formulation of a disaster plan. Many companies have a disaster plan which has been devised by the safety committee. This should be revised and updated at least yearly, with the nurse's involvement. The goals of a disaster plan are to prevent or minimize injuries and deaths of workers and residents, to minimize property damage, effectively triage, and facilitate the resumption of necessary business activities (Ossler 1992). The simplest and most effective disaster plan is a poster illustrating the map of each level of the plant, with instructions for reaching the telephone, calling for assistance, shutting down any machinery, maintaining clear exits and evacuating an injured worker or all building occupants. It is important that the nurse be familiar with the plan, as in many cases, the nurse will be on site before anyone has called for outside help or begun to prepare for evacuation. All company employees should be given an opportunity to familiarize themselves with the plan, and each division or section of the plant should conduct periodic rehearsals, either physically or verbally, for the allocation of roles in the case of an emergency situation.

Secondary prevention

Secondary prevention in the work place consists of primary care provided to injured or ill workers and screening for known work place hazards. According to Ossler (1992) interventions should always focus on designing the health hazard out of the work. In the case of a chemical hazard, this may include substituting a less toxic chemical, isolating the chemical in the work process or isolating the worker from the chemical. For physical hazards such as protracted periods of work at a video display terminal (VDT) intervention may include redesigning the desk, chair and lighting, providing appropriate rest breaks, exercises and relaxation strategies, and ongoing assessment of the worker. Environmental concerns should be reported to the company manager with recommendations for alternatives (Ossler 1992).

Many non-occupational illnesses are treated in the work place; for example, upper respiratory infections and simple gastrointestinal ailments. Among the occupational illnesses arising, some may be acute, such as allergic skin reactions to work place chemicals; or chronic, such as respiratory impairment. Some illnesses are difficult to categorize as occupational or non-occupational. For example, due to the long latency period of some carcinomas, symptoms do not occur until long after the exposure. It is very difficult, therefore, to attribute a causal association between carcinogenic substances in the work place and the development of the disease (Ray 1985). In addition, some occupational illnesses are a result of interactive effects. For example, chemical exposure to metals used in welding may combine with a lifetime of smoking and living in a chemically polluted environment to produce lung cancer. This makes delineation of the relative risk of each factor difficult.

Occupational injuries are specific to the industry. In industries which use heavy equipment, back injuries are common, as are strains, sprains or crushing injuries. Where there is excessive heat, heat exhaustion may occur. In companies where chemicals are handled, employees are at risk for toxic reactions, burns or inhalation injuries. Some industries have a high incidence of laceration, such as results from handling glass in a bottling operation, or metal in machinery shops. Employees engaged in repetitive packaging or keyboard work are at risk for overuse syndrome, often diagnosed as tenosynovitis. Those working on computer terminals also may be prone to eye strain and/or shoulder pain. Many and varied jobs produce headaches, fatigue and stress disorders.

Because primary care for the ill or injured worker is planned, implemented and evaluated based on a thorough assessment of the worker as well as the precipitating situation, the occupational health nurse must be skilled in physical assessment, triage, first aid, crisis intervention and counselling.

Depending upon the extent of occupational health facilities, treatment, guidance and counselling may be provided at the worksite, or the worker may be referred for more extensive or specialized care. External community resources for care include physicians, physiotherapists, medical specialists, family counsellors, or community agencies providing services for a range of needs.

Many cases requiring counselling and/or referral involve situations where the stress of work has exacerbated or accelerated a non-occupational condition. For example, the worker undergoing stress-related problems such as family illness, marital breakdown, parenting problems or substance abuse often has a difficult time coping at work. Such individuals may be preoccupied with personal problems, engage in self-destructive behaviours, perform inadequately on the job, and occasionally present a safety hazard to those working around them. Some seek refuge in abusing alcohol or other substances, placing themselves and their co-workers at risk. Others vent their frustration by engaging in erratic behaviour, taking their problems out on others around them and interfering with the disciplined functioning of the job. To provide assistance to these workers, the nurse may conduct an initial assessment, then make a referral to a community resource. In other cases, where trust has been established and the employee's needs are not beyond the nurse's capabilities, the nurse and the worker will plan a series of counselling sessions to explore the problem and generate possible solutions.

Some community resources provide inhouse services to the work place. For example, in many locations, the local alcohol and drug authority will provide an employee assistance program to help workers with chemical dependencies. Other agencies provide smoking cessation classes, fitness and lifestyle classes and stress management programs. In some cases, counselling is provided outside the work place; for example, for marital or family counselling. Depending upon the employee's wishes, the occupational health nurse may liaise with the counsellor, or follow the employee's progress by maintaining ongoing dialogue with the employee.

Management of illnesses and injuries often depends upon whether the nurse has sole responsibility for the occupational health centre, or whether there is a physician in attendance. In many cases, the nurse is responsible for the centre, with a physician attending at regular intervals, such as once or twice weekly. In other cases, the nurse conducts the occupational health practice with a physician from outside the company contracted to see workers when necessary, and to provide physician back-up for nursing recommendations. In very large industries, there may be a physician on duty at all times. Occasionally, the occupational health nurse will be employed by one or more small companies on a contractual basis. In these situations, the nurse conducts follow up of illnesses and injuries which have occurred in his or her absence, maintaining an accurate record of events.

Careful documentation of each case is necessary to evaluate outcomes of treatment and, as mentioned previously, for the analysis of work place hazards. In addition, many work place injuries are referred for compensation, through local worker's compensation boards. In such cases, the recording of the events surrounding the injury and treatment strategies undertaken must be available for review. Confidentiality of all health records must be maintained, however, statistics on the incidence and prevalence of illnesses and injuries may be made available to the health and safety committee, management and employee groups, as an indication of the effectiveness of health and safety promotion strategies.

Tertiary prevention

The object of tertiary prevention activities in the work place is to promote adherence to regimens for rehabilitation, and to minimize occupational hazards. Injury impacts will be influenced by job and labour market characteristics, the nature of informal family and community support networks and a range of other factors (Quinlan & Bohle 1991). The nurse can facilitate rehabilitation programs by contributing to the development of a company health and rehabilitation policy which includes guidelines for return to work of the ill or injured worker and for monitoring, improving and maintaining plant safety.

In some cases, the nurse may visit the ill or injured worker in the hospital or home before his or her return to work. At this time, the rehabilitation program can be discussed, and a realistic schedule planned. Many men, in particular, return to the work place following a heart attack, or heart surgery. They may be apprehensive about their capabilities, the threat of work causing further damage to their heart, or the attitudes of co-workers. A home visit can provide reassurance that they will be allowed to ease back into the job in stages, and that there will be support and assistance available in the work place if necessary. In cases where there are two or more employees debilitated by the same condition, a peer support program may be instituted. This can be as formal or informal as the employees prefer, with the nurse being fully involved, or acting only as the catalyst to self-help.

Most employees returning to work following either illness or injury are also reassured if the occupational health nurse establishes contact with their physician and/or the community health nurse who may be involved with the case. The occupational health nurse can act as liaison, communicating the job characteristics to the physician and/or community health nurse, while ensuring that the physician's prescribed schedule of activity for the worker can be adhered to.

The field of occupational health nursing is rapidly advancing, with the current focus on wellness, and the recognition that for those employed, one-third of their time is spent in the world of work. Occupational health nursing is a special area of nursing challenge: one in which the community is a captive group of well and functioning individuals engaged in the normal activities of the work place. To promote and maintain continuing wellness in this environment requires a dedication to the ideology of primary health care; competent nursing skills; a knowledge of the world at large, complemented by strong written and verbal communication skills; and the independence of thought to adopt an advocacy role for all members and all levels of the occupational community.

REMOTE AREA NURSING

Perhaps the most appropriate standard bearer of primary health care is the remote area nurse (RAN), for it is in the remote nursing situation that the nurse assumes sole responsibility for providing comprehensive health care for all community residents in the place where they live and work. As the primary caregiver, the nurse must function as the representative of all sectors involved in contributing to community health, including the political, economic, environmental, religious, cultural, education and health sectors. Potts (1990) describes remote area nursing as revolving around antenatal care, child health, immunization, school health, sexually transmitted diseases, the Royal Flying Doctor services, community education and illness prevention.

Most RANs live in their work environment, usually a nursing station, and most are on call to community residents on a 24-hour-a-day basis. With no physical or psychological respite from practice, the nurse must rely on personal strengths and self-sufficiency to maintain a sense of perspective. According to Harris (1991, p. 103), many RANs survive on 'the gift of the gab and guts'. The role requires an independent spirit, confidence in one's clinical and interpersonal capabilities, extraordinary resourcefulness, caring and commitment to helping the isolated community and an appreciation of the cultural factors which render each community unique. Clearly, the nurse must adopt a non-ethnocentric approach in order to be sensitive to value systems which may differ considerably from her or his own. Bushy (1992) identifies common values which seem to pervade most rural communities. These include 'adhering to traditional gender role behaviour and demonstrating stoic self-sufficiency' (p. 345). In her view, nurses must be knowledgeable of these values as well as of their impact on families and community health and health behaviour.

Harris (1991) suggests that 'once you have been in a community for a while you feel like you are part of the family' (p. 102). However, this closeness with the community can be both rewarding and difficult for the nurse. For example, issues such as sexual assault in a small community may divide citizens into those who say guilty and those who say not guilty and the nurse who is trying to advocate for both perpetrator and victim (Harris 1991). Harris cites a case where she notified the authorities of a child who had been physically abused and was herself abused in the street and had rocks and bottles thrown at her dogs as a result. Most nurses endure violence at some time or other during their remote area nursing experience yet remain dedicated to helping the community.

As co-ordinator of primary health care to the remote community, the nurse functions as an advocate for the community and for the individuals and families who live and work there. Remote area nursing thus incorporates the role of family and child health nurse, school health nurse, and mental health nurse.

Primary prevention

Managing health promotion and illness prevention within an isolated community can be both rewarding and intimidating. Despite the frustration of encountering what are usually inadequate resources and sporadic back-up services, there are rewards in the recognition that many positive health gains in the community are a direct result of nursing efforts.

Health education is a major aspect of the role. Nurses in remote communities rarely have the time or resources to develop and conduct community-wide health promotion campaigns, and thus devote a considerable portion of their family visits, whether in clinic or home, to educating parents about child development, nutrition, family planning or health protection practices. Some health education activities are aimed at facilitating the mental health of community members. This may include using the local media (posters in the school, community newspaper) to heighten community awareness of mental health issues and/or teaching stress and coping techniques on an individual or group basis. The local school usually provides a forum for community collaboration on a range of topics. In many cases, the nurse collaborates with the teacher(s) on health promotion campaigns related to nutrition, sexual health and AIDS awareness, alcohol and other substance abuse and smoking prevention. In addition, the nurse may be called upon to teach community members such health protective behaviours as cardiopulmonary resuscitation and to monitor the community's water and sewage systems as well as any hazards present in the environment.

In many remote communities, the population is primarily composed of indigenous people. Historically, one of the obstacles to effective health education has been that the goals and objectives of health care for these people have been determined from a model of health appropriate to those who administer their health care in distant urban environments. The outcome of such arrangements has been health care which is neither holistic nor culturally relevant to those for whom it was intended. It is often the RAN who attempts to rectify this situation by instigating the return of health care to the culture and by helping to mobilize community members to take an active part in health promotion and health education.

As community advocate the RAN serves as communications intermediary between the community and the outside world, including the health care system. To perform this role, the nurse needs to learn the local principles of communication and the social organization patterns (Hagey & Buller 1983). Communication principles include the people's learning styles, such as whether they are more receptive to written, pictorial or verbal (perhaps story telling) communication. Included also, are local cultural metaphors and customs for teaching (Hagey & Buller 1983). Some cultures place great emphasis on their particular rules of speech; for example, the use of silence and ambiguous responses, while others are more concerned with social distance and the posturing which accompanies communication. In all communities it takes a while for the nurse to encounter a wide enough range of interactions to feel confident that the norms and conventions are being upheld. In many remote area nursing posts this process can be made easier by discussing the formal and informal rules with nurses who have been in the area previously. Von Sturmer's (1981) insightful explanation of the do's and don'ts of talking with Aborigines is recommended for further reading on this topic.

Patterns of social organization which the nurse must become familiar with include the authority relationships, rituals and customs of the people. For example, the traditional healers in native cultures often represent the ultimate health care medium (Reser 1991). The traditional healer is the symbol of an earlier holistic health care system which is only very recently being retrieved. In the past, traditional healing emphasized the unity of the person, society, nature and the supernatural, and the healer was a multifaceted practitioner who acted on a number of religious, medical and social issues (Hodgson 1982). The influence of the traditional healer has, to date, been an untapped resource to the RAN. However, nurses are now beginning to collaborate with the healers to explore ways in which they can work together within the community to deliver more comprehensive care, and to make health education more meaningful within the cultural context (Gregory & Stewart 1987).

Some of the health education topics that are important in indigenous communities include stress management and attending to the personal development of the local people. In many cases where one culture has been frustrated by enforced assimilation into another culture, there is a need to prevent demoralization by nurturing a sense of self-esteem. This can be helped by encouraging self-expression through creative outlets; for example, painting or music. Establishing and supporting projects and programs which contribute to self-development are important strategies for facilitating mental health in the community.

Secondary prevention

The health issues confronting the RAN include most of those occurring in any community, with additional challenges related to isolation and/or the uniqueness of working with indigenous people. Because of the isolation, treatment for illness or injury may be less than optimal, with the nurse attempting to fill the gap left by the lack of medical resources and welfare services. In addition to being responsible for handling emergencies and providing primary care, it is up to the nurse to discriminate between those who can be safely treated at the nursing station and those who must be evacuated. The impact of this is compounded by the responsibility of maintaining links with the outside world through what are often erratic and fragile means of communication, and interacting in sometimes violent situations (Cramer 1987). In an Australian survey of RAN practice, many RANs expressed concern about the lack of protocols and guidelines for nursing practice which often has a substantial medical responsibility (Kreger 1991). Kreger's report identified the need for ongoing education which could be accessed by nurses in remote areas. One useful educational strategy has been the development of a remote area nursing orientation manual which describes many commonly encountered situations and treatment strategies used by RANs currently in practice (Menere 1992).

Case finding and case management is an unending challenge varying from situation to situation. Many childbirth complications are caused by malnutrition and a lack of antenatal care. In many remote areas, births frequently occur outside of institutions with inadequate access to facilities for emergency care. In addition to midwifery services, the nurse can provide clear instructions and guidance to the family on caring for the mother and child, encouraging postnatal follow up. In cases where the mother has given birth outside the community and where there has been little medical follow up the nurse is required to provide extended monitoring and guidance.

The difficulties of providing primary care in isolated communities are compounded in Aboriginal communities, as Aboriginal people have a higher than average rate of childbirth complications and perinatal death from disease and infection (Thomson & Briscoe 1992). Secondary intervention for diseases and infections can be facilitated by early case finding and treatment. In some cases, the nurse will provide treatment according to a departmental or agency protocol for recurring types of illnesses; on other occasions, it will be up to the nurse to obtain medical advice and assistance on an individual basis.

Another area of particular concern in Aboriginal communities is the treatment of alcohol-related problems. In dealing with Aboriginal groups a community approach is often most effective. Bain (1974) suggests that many Aborigines drink because of group pressure. The collective nature of the drinking act thus precludes moderation and refusal. According to Bryant and Carroll (1978), because Aboriginals become alcoholics in groups they should be treated in groups rather than in the way of white people who become alcoholics one by one. Brady (1991) cites Gibson, an anthropologist, who adds an interesting insight into the problem of alcohol abuse in Aboriginal communities. He argues that for too long Aboriginal society has accepted that the social phenomenon of alcohol among the young is the expression of culture and identity. He makes the point that the drinker who spends the family's money on alcohol and who can be heard explaining his kinship ties to his fellows as they drink, is denying and distorting true Aboriginal tradition to the point of exploitation. He suggests that it is time to stop interpreting alcoholism as some kind of helpless result of culture clash. Similarly, he urges that we stop seeing gambling as some kind of traditional redistribution of wealth and confront these issues in a non-exploitative but useful way (Gibson, in Brady 1991). Clearly, the most helpful approach to the problem is one which is culturally sensitive yet is aimed at the individual problem and circumstances.

In some communities, poverty combined with the pervasive sense of helplessness and frustration enhanced by alcohol abuse produces a high incidence of violence (Mardiros 1987). This may take the form of child or spouse abuse, homicide, suicide or violent acts which, on occasion, are committed against the nurse. It is sometimes difficult to remain in the advocacy role in the face of violence, however, help must be obtained for all members of the family or community. Immediate crisis intervention involves reassurance, providing a safe refuge if possible, and initiating a program of counselling. This may be thwarted in some cases however, by the transient nature of either the victim or perpetrator, or the unwillingness of either to engage in setting long term goals for change, particularly in the case of spouse and/or alcohol abuse.

Other health problems presented to the remote area nurse include lifestyle-related conditions such as obesity, dental caries, cardiovascular disease and diabetes. The need for nutrition and general health counselling persists across primary, secondary and tertiary prevention strategies. A difficulty which many nurses face when treating residents in the remote areas is that of reaching the ill or injured client. When a home visit is made, the nurse's vehicle must be equipped with survival supplies, tools, maps, weather forecasts, current information on road conditions and transportation schedules, creating the extraordinary demand that nursing skills be supplemented by a working knowledge of advanced information processing, navigation and automechanics.

Being removed from the administration of services to the remote area makes it difficult for the nurse to exert political pressure on those with the power to improve sanitation, housing and sewage. However, many nurses attempt to overcome this by persistent written communication outlining the health hazards in the community, suggesting improvements to the health authorities and lobbying government officials. A further strategy, and one which contributes to professional networking, is to document the conditions for publication in nursing or allied health journals.

Tertiary prevention

Rehabilitation of the ill or injured remote community resident is very often the sole responsibility of the nurse. Those with chronic illness, such as cancer, diabetes and heart conditions, must be continuously monitored and evaluated in order to revise plans or strategies for care. The rehabilitation of those suffering from alcohol and drug abuse presents a particular problem.

The key to restoring such individuals to a normal lifestyle is often a program in which physical health is restored, new styles of coping are suggested, and a behavioural substitute for the substance is offered. Learning a new skill or developing a creative hobby can be most helpful. In instituting programs for change, the significant value of peer support must be considered. Behaviour change can be more optimistically expected if an informal self-help group can be arranged to reinforce each member's positive efforts and to strengthen the resolve to abandon or reduce consumption of the offending substance.

The remote area nurse also assumes responsibility for the convalescing injured individual. In all cases, careful recording of treatment, care and progress must be done, in order to evaluate outcomes and fulfil reporting requirements. The task of documentation is often considered the most distasteful aspect of remote area nursing. However, when practice is conducted in what is often a precarious balance between professional approval and the needs of the population, it is best to have the legal protection of a meticulous record of nursing activities.

The single most powerful tool the nurse can use to influence a community's health is the ability to portray a positive role model for healthy living. In addition to this, the nurse must be manager, practitioner, social support system, political activist and friend to the community she or he serves; working out the balance between over involvement and enough participation to be effective (Hodgson 1982). Most importantly, the nurse must be able to view life through the eyes of another culture without abandoning or feeling apologetic for his or her own culture (Stewart et al 1985).

SUMMARY

Many community health nurses practise in situations which extend the generalist orientation to specialized roles. This chapter has discussed several of these roles: the child health role, the community mental health role, the school health role, the occupational health and remote area nursing roles. Each has unique knowledge and skills which correspond to the requirements of practice in their respective settings. However, in defining their role according to the concepts, values and commitment to primary health care, nurses practising within these and other community health nursing specialties maintain a unified approach to the attainment of health for all communities.

Study exercises

---

1. You are conducting a developmental assessment on a 2-year-old child. The mother confides to you that her mother (who lives in the family home) and her husband are constantly bickering about the child's development (toilet training, discipline, foods). How would you guide her?

2. Some social researchers claim that the trend towards deinstitutionalization of the mentally ill has had a negative effect in that it has swelled the numbers of homeless and alienated many people from society. What are the two sides of this argument?
3. Identify the steps you would take if you were the school health nurse and a teacher revealed to you that she suspected child sexual abuse in one of her students, a 12-year-old girl.
4. Provide a persuasive argument for instituting a quit smoking campaign in a heavy metal industry.
5. Explain how you would institute a program for primary, secondary and tertiary prevention in dealing with alcohol abuse in a remote community.

REFERENCES

AOHNA 1991 Occupational health nursing in Australia: a guide to employment. Australian Occupational Health Nurses Association, Melbourne

Bain M 1974 Alcohol use and traditional social control in Aboriginal society. In: Hetzel B (ed) Better health for Aborigines? University of Queensland Press, St Lucia

Bajnok I 1988 Specialization meets entry to practice. The Canadian Nurse 84(6):23-24

Baumgart A 1988 Called to account—nursing education for yesterday or tomorrow. Proceedings of the Olive Anstey International Nursing Conference, Perth, pp 1.07-1.15

Beckman Blomquist K 1992 Health promotion through nutrition, exercise and sleep. In: Stanhope M, Lancaster J (eds) Community health nursing: process and practice for promoting health 3rd edn. C V Mosby, St Louis, pp 592-611

Benner P 1984 From novice to expert: excellence and power in clinical nursing practice. Addison-Wesley, Menlo Park

Berger K 1983 The developing person through the lifespan. Worth, New York

Berns J, Hamilton M 1985 Nursing role in community mental health. In: Jarvis L (ed) Community health nursing: keeping the public healthy, 2nd edn. F A Davis, Philadelphia, pp 445-478

Blank Sherman J, Alexander M, Gomez D, Kim M, Marole P 1992 Intervention program for obese school children. Journal of Community Health Nursing 9(3):183-190

Boyer D, Heppner I 1992 Community mental health: problem identification and treatment. In: Stanhope M, Lancaster J Community health nursing: process and practice for promoting health 3rd edn. C V Mosby, St Louis, pp 351-364

Bradshaw M 1988 Nursing of the family in health and illness: a developmental approach. Appleton & Lange, Norwalk

Brady M 1991 Drug and alcohol use among Aboriginal people. In: Reid J, Trompf P The health of Aboriginal Australia. Harcourt Brace Jovanovich, Sydney, pp 173-217

Bryant V, Carroll J 1978 Aboriginal alcoholism—where are we going? White man's way or black man's way? Aboriginal Health Worker 11(2):20-21

Burdekin B, Carter J, Dethlefs W 1989 Our homeless children. Report of the national inquiry into homeless children. Australian Government Publishing Service, Canberra

Bushy A 1992 Rural determinants in family health: considerations for community nurses. In: Saucier K (ed) Perspectives in family and community health. C V Mosby, St Louis, pp 340-346

Clark M 1984 Community nursing for today and tomorrow. Reston Publishing, Reston

Cramer J 1987 A blind eye: community health services in remote areas of Australia. Community Health Studies XI(2):135-138

Commonwealth of Australia 1992 National Mental Health Policy. Australian Government Publishing Service, Canberra

Commonwealth-State Council on Non-English Speaking Background Women's Issues 1991 The National Non-English Speaking Background Women's Health Strategy. Australian Government Publishing Service, Canberra

Dickenson-Hazard N 1988 School-age children and adolescents. In: Stanhope M, Lancaster J (eds) Community health nursing: process and practice for promoting health, 2nd edn. C V Mosby, St Louis, pp 442-474

Dickenson-Hazard N 1992 School-age children and adolescents. In: Stanhope M, Lancaster J (eds) Community health nursing : process and practice for promoting health, 3rd edn. C V Mosby, St Louis, pp 485-511

Gregory D, Stewart P 1987 Nurses and traditional healers: now is the time to speak. The Canadian Nurse 83(8):25-27

Hagey R, Buller E 1983 Drumming and dancing: a new rhythm in nursing care. The Canadian Nurse 79(4):28-31

Harris M 1991 The day to day life of a remote area nurse. Proceedings, Development and Diversity: Remote and Rural Primary Health Care Conference, 25-26 July, The University of Sydney Cumberland College of Health Sciences, Sydney, pp 99-106

Hodgson C 1982 Ambiguity and paradox in outpost nursing. International Nursing Review 29(4):108-117

Holzemer W 1992 Linking primary health care and self-care through case management. International Nursing Review 39(3):83-89

Igoe J, Speer S 1992 The community health nurse in the schools. In: Stanhope M, Lancaster J (eds) Community health nursing: process and practice for promoting health, 3rd edn. C V Mosby, St Louis, pp 707-730

Jorm A 1987 Sex and age differences in depression: a quantitative synthesis of published research. Australian and New Zealand Journal of Psychiatry 21:46-53

Kreger A 1991 Remote area nursing practice: a question of education. Council of Remote Area Nurses of Australia, Perth

Kristein M 1982 The economics of health promotion at the worksite. Health Education Quarterly 9 (Suppl):27-36

Lancaster J, Kerschner D 1988 Community mental health: problem, identification, prevention and intervention. In: Stanhope M, Lancaster J (eds) Community health nursing: process and practice for promoting health, 2nd edn. C V Mosby, St Louis, pp 629-648

McMurray A 1991 Expertise in community health nursing. Unpublished Doctoral Thesis. Department of Education, The University of Western Australia, Perth

McMurray A 1992 Influences on parent-child relationships in non-custodial mothers. Australian Journal of Marriage & Family, 13(3):138-147

Mardiros M 1987 Primary health care and Canada's indigenous people. The Canadian Nurse 83(8):25-27

Menere R 1992 Remote area nursing orientation manual. Faculty of Health Sciences, University of New England, Lismore

National Health & Medical Research Council 1991 Women and mental health. Monograph Series No.1 Australian Government Publishing Service, Canberra

National Occupational Health and Safety Commission 1988 Asbestos—code of practice and guidance notes. National Occupational Health and Safety Commission, Australian Government Publishing Service, Canberra

Oda D 1985 Community health nursing in innovative school health roles and programs. In: Archer S, Fleshman R (eds) Community health nursing, 3rd edn. Wadsworth, Monterey, pp 368-393

Ossler C 1988 The community health nurse in occupational health. In: Stanhope M, Lancaster J (eds) Community health nursing: process and practice for promoting health, 2nd edn. C V Mosby, St Louis, 791-804

Ossler C 1992 The community health nurse in occupational health. In: Stanhope M, Lancaster J (eds) Community health nursing: process and practice for promoting health, 3rd edn. C V Mosby, St Louis, pp 731-746

Parsons M, Felton G 1992 Role performance and job satisfaction of school nurses. Western Journal of Nursing Research 14(4):498-511

Porter P 1985 Community health nurses in community mental health. In: Archer S, Fleshman R (eds) Community health nursing, 3rd edn. Wadsworth, Monterey, pp 352-367

Potts P 1990 Pretty rugged in the outback. The Australian Nurses Journal 19(9):13-14

Quinlan M, Bohle P 1991 Managing occupational health and safety in Australia: a multidisciplinary approach. MacMillan Co, Melbourne

Ray L 1985 Community health nursing at the worksite. In: Archer S, Fleshman R (eds) Community health nursing, 3rd edn. Wadsworth, Monterey, pp 394-417

Reser J 1991 Aboriginal mental health: conflicting cultural perspectives In: Reid J, Trompf P (eds) The health of Aboriginal Australia. Harcourt Brace Jovanovich, Sydney, pp 218-291

Schofield T 1992 Health promotion in primary care—does teamwork make a difference? Journal of Interprofessional Care 6(2):97-101

Sebastian J 1992 Vulnerable populations in the community. In: M Stanhope, J Lancaster (eds) Community health nursing: process and practice for promoting health, 3rd edn. C V Mosby, St Louis, pp 365-390

Shepherd R 1986 Economic benefits of enhanced fitness. Kinetics Publishers, Champaign, Illinois

Stewart M, Searl S, Smillie C, May R, Sayers A 1985 Specialized nursing roles in unique community-based settings. In: Stewart M (ed) Community health nursing in Canada. Gage, Toronto, pp 179-193

Thomson N, Briscoe N 1992 Overview of Aboriginal health status in Western Australia. Australian Government Publishing Service, Canberra

Von Sturmer J 1981 Talking with Aborigines. Australian Institute of Aboriginal Studies Newsletter. New Series no. 15, March, Canberra

Winkleby M, Rockhill B, Jatulis D, S 1992 The medical origin of homelessness. American Journal of Public Health 82(10):1394-1398

Withrow C 1988 The community health nurse in the schools. In: Stanhope M, Lancaster J (eds) Community health nursing: process and practice for promoting health, 2nd edn. C V Mosby, St Louis, pp 779-790

PART 2

From theory to practice

INTRODUCTION

The development of nursing as a scientific discipline has been primarily dependent on the accumulation of professional knowledge. The domain of nursing knowledge thus represents a perspective which is based on an evolving philosophy and history, former practice, theory, research, and emerging ideas of nursing scholars (Kenney 1990). To date, the collective wisdom which informs this knowledge domain addresses nursing concepts and problems, the processes and tools for assessment, diagnosis, intervention and evaluation, and research designs and methods which are congruent with professional goals (Meleis 1985). Nursing models guide this type of inquiry and the process of organizing knowledge within the nursing domain. The nursing process, which was first documented by Yura and Walsh in 1967 and which continues to be refined and reformulated, provides a framework for linking the conceptual models of nursing with the realities of clinical practice. This section provides an overview of some of the more commonly used nursing models in Chapter 3 and an examination of how the nursing process can be applied to community health nursing in Chapter 4.

Content: Part 2

3. Conceptual models for practice

Terminology
Nursing models
   Systems: the Neuman health care systems model
   Adaptation: the Roy adaptation model
   Self-care: Orem's self-care nursing model
   Health promotion: Pender's health promotion model
   Other models and theories
   Family theories

4. The process of nursing in the community

The nursing process
The nursing process in community health nursing practice
   Assessment
      Data gathering
      Organization of data
      Cultural assessment
      Analysis
   Nursing diagnosis
   Planning
      Rumba?
   Implementation
      Resources
      Referral
         The decision to refer
   Evaluation
   Discharge planning

3. Conceptual models for practice

Professional nursing practice is grounded in a theoretical foundation. Theoretical concepts are developed as nursing practice evolves and is examined with respect to existing knowledge. When these concepts are scientifically validated in a multitude of practice situations, they provide guidelines for practice by way of conceptual models. Conceptual models attempt to explain the nursing paradigm, or overall scheme, which relates the nursing client to the context or environment of care, to the health or illness situation, and to the practice of nursing. Because each model has its own explanation for the nursing paradigm, some are more appropriate to community health nursing than others. This chapter discusses four such models and provides a comment on the suitability of others as a guide to nursing the family and community. Before discussing particular models, some clarification of terminology may be helpful.

TERMINOLOGY

A *hypothesis* or proposition specifies the relationship between two or more concepts or ideas. Hypotheses are derived from observing and reflecting on patterns of meanings in communication during social interaction such as occurs during nurse-client encounters (Aamodt 1991). When hypotheses have been empirically tested through research in many settings, they may be woven into a theory. A *theory* is thus a logically interconnected set of confirmed hypotheses or propositions (McKay 1986). A *conceptual model* can then be constructed to explain theory and the ideas which comprise it. Conceptual models can therefore be thought of as symbolic 'maps' or structures which integrate the concepts and ideas of a theory into a meaningful configuration. The term *paradigm* is usually used to encapsulate the total universe of concern; that is, a profession's theories, concepts and models. Some theorists refer to the nursing paradigm as a *metaparadigm* (Whall & Fawcett 1991). Because both terms express the global perspective of an all-encompassing knowledge base, the choice of expression is arbitrary.

Conceptual models are of value to nursing in that they represent a tool to link theory and practice; they help to clarify thinking about the elements of a practice situation and their relationship to one another; they help practitioners of nursing to communicate with one another in a meaningful way, and they serve as a guide to practice, education and research (McFarlane 1986). The choice of model determines the kind of information that will be gathered and the way it will be organized and interpreted. Because of the uniqueness and scope of the information required for community health nursing, certain models serve as a more appropriate community practice guide than others; for example, Neuman's health care systems model; Roy's adaptation model; Orem's self-care nursing model, and Pender's health promotion model.

NURSING MODELS

Nursing models can be categorized according to their primary focus. For example, interaction models focus on the nature of the nurse-client interaction; developmental models focus on theories of development or change to explain a nursing situation; and systems models use general systems theory as a basis for describing elements of a nursing situation (McFarlane 1986).

Each model attempts to explain the nursing paradigm according to its particular tenets but all are structured around defining the four major theoretical elements of nursing theory: person, environment, health and nursing. Those with the greatest application to community health nursing are those in which people are viewed in the context of a larger macrostructure or system. The individual is seen as being in continuous interaction with the environment or community. The community can be seen as having either a facilitative or disruptive influence on health, health care and the change process. The nursing goal common to each model is to assess, plan, implement and evaluate ways to make the community a healthy place to live, one in which recipients of care can be assisted to assume personal responsibility for their health (Lee & Lancaster 1988).

Systems: the Neuman health care systems model

A system is defined by Rapaport (1968) as a 'whole which functions as a whole by virtue of the interdependence of its parts' (p. 4). The openness of a system refers to the extent to which its boundaries are open and energy is exchanged between the system and the environment. In a closed system, no energy is exchanged (Lee & Lancaster 1988).

The health care system is an open system in that there is a continuous flow of input, throughput (process), output and feedback. In repeated cycles, the input, process and output become feedback for further input. Neuman (1982, 1989) explains that, in this pattern, the system can be seen as moving towards differentiation and elaboration for further growth and survival. In other words, the system becomes refined for specific functions.

Neuman's health care systems model is derived from the general systems theory of Bertalanffy (1952). According to systems theory, the whole is conceptualized in terms of its interacting elements, somewhat like a mobile. As illustrated in Chapter 4: when one part is touched, there is a reverberation to other parts. Neuman's model is an open systems model of two key components: stress and reaction to it. Both noxious and beneficial stressors operate on the system which attempts to maintain balance or homeostasis. Once the balance is disrupted, energy is expended to cope. This can take the form of 'entropy', where the energy flow moves towards extinction by general disorganization, randomness and dissipation of energy; or 'negentropy' (evolution), where energy is absorbed so that the system can increase its organization and complexity to develop towards a steady state (Neuman 1982, 1989). The family provides an example of this. Chaotic families would demonstrate entropy, whereas energized, egalitarian families could be described as 'negentropic' (see Ch. 4).

Person or client

The person or client in the Neuman model is a composite of the relationship between physiologic, psychologic, sociocultural and developmental variables (Neuman 1982, 1989).

Environment

The environment includes all internal and external forces surrounding an individual at any point in time, and varying according to needs. This includes all factors affecting and affected by the system.

Health

Health or wellness is seen as a condition in which all parts or subparts are in harmony with the whole individual. In other words, there are no disruptive needs. Disharmony due to disruptive needs reduces the state of wellness.

Nursing

Nursing is an interdependent part of the health care system and its surrounding social system. Nursing's reciprocal relationship with system subparts contributes to optimal functioning and the evolutionary survival of the whole system. The nurse assesses the two processes of entropy and negentropy to guide her or his interventions, which aim to counteract entropy with a form of evolutionary adaptation, restoring and maintaining equilibrium between forces or stressors. The nurse assesses the factors which influence a person's perceptual field; the meaning a stressor has to the client (validated by the client); and the factors in his or her own perceptual field which influence assessment and care giving (Neuman 1982, 1989).

As illustrated in Figure 3.1, the model is represented by a series of concentric rings surrounding a central core consisting of basic survival factors common to all. The concentric rings vary in size and distance from

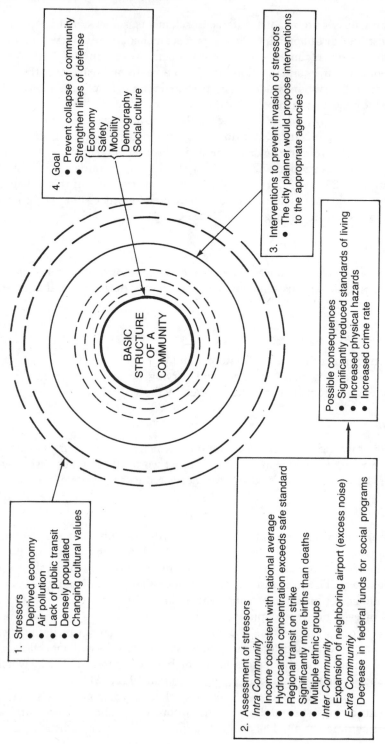

4. Goal
   • Prevent collapse of community
   • Strengthen lines of defense
     Economy
     Safety
     Mobility
     Demography
     Social culture

3. Interventions to prevent invasion of stressors
   • The city planner would propose interventions
     to the appropriate agencies

Possible consequences
   • Significantly reduced standards of living
   • Increased physical hazards
   • Increased crime rate

BASIC
STRUCTURE
OF A
COMMUNITY

1. Stressors
   • Deprived economy
   • Air pollution
   • Lack of public transit
   • Densely populated
   • Changing cultural values

2. Assessment of stressors
   Intra Community
   • Income consistent with national average
   • Hydrocarbon concentration exceeds safe standard
   • Regional transit on strike
   • Significantly more births than deaths
   • Multiple ethnic groups
   Inter Community
   • Expansion of neighboring airport (excess noise)
   Extra Community
   • Decrease in federal funds for social programs

Fig. 3.1 The Neuman health care systems model (Copyright B. Neuman 1970).

the centre. These make up the flexible lines of resistance. Stressors have the potential to temporarily incapacitate an individual or possibly reduce her or his internal lines of resistance which protect the core structure. This state of resistance varies over time, and from one individual to another. The outer broken ring, the flexible line of defence, is a protective buffer to prevent stressors breaking through the solid line of defence (Neuman 1982, 1989).

The community

Neuman's model is ideally suited to guide community health nursing. The central core of survival factors in a community consists of the physical structure, locale, community history, and age, race and sex composition of the population (Clark 1984). The lines of resistance represent such things as available health care, the educational level of community members, adequacy of transportation, recreational facilities and immunization levels of the population. The normal line of defence would be the presence and adequacy of protective services, general nutritional and income levels, the adequacy of housing and community attitudes toward health. The flexible line of defence would include the availability of health care funding, employment levels and climate (Clark 1984).

Assessment of the community as part of a larger system involves assessing intracommunity factors, that is forces occurring within a community; intercommunity factors, that is forces occurring between one or more communities and extracommunity factors which occur outside of the community but in some way impact on the community (Benedict & Behringer Sproles 1982). As indicated in Figure 3.1, primary prevention would involve preventing the invasion of stressors and strengthening the lines of defence to prevent the collapse of the community.

For example, to strengthen the lines of resistance against social isolation of the elderly, a community day care program may be instituted. Secondary prevention would involve home visits and activities designed to help those who may be suffering from neglect or abuse, thus strengthening the normal line of defence. Tertiary prevention would aim at strengthening the flexible line of defence by instituting follow-up programs of care for those requiring assistance and by allocating community funds for ongoing programs of prevention and care. Because of the community's interdependence on its subsystems (in this case, the ageing family subsystem), strengthening the subsystem strengthens the central core of the community, thus moving the system towards homeostasis.

Neuman's systems model also provides a useful guide for planning family nursing care. Reed (1989, 1993) suggests that the family's primary, secondary and tertiary stressors must be assessed as well as the extent to which the family's line of defence has been penetrated. Examples of factors which influence the family's flexible line of defence include their capacity for role enactment, rule implementation, decision making mechanisms, task-allocation processes and bonding patterns. Primary stressors may include

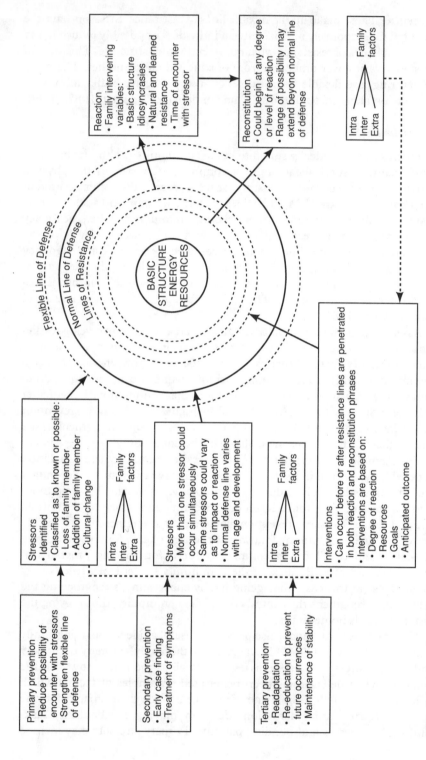

Fig. 3.2 Adaptation of Neuman model approach to viewing family problems (From Neuman 1982).

career change, marriage, and entry of children into the system. Unemployment, disasters, death of a family member and marriage difficulties would be examples of secondary stressors. Tertiary stressors include such things as substance abuse, chronic physical or mental illness, loss of body functioning or divorce. Reed (1989, 1993) proposes that once the family's stressors are identified, primary, secondary and tertiary intervention strategies can be planned to restore the family system to its functional capacity, as illustrated in Figure 3.2.

Adaptation: the Roy adaptation model

The Roy adaptation model is primarily a systems model with interactionist levels of analysis. According to Roy (1980), the model views the person or client as having elements linked together in such a way that force on the linkages can be increased or decreased. Increased force or tension comes from strains within the system or from the environment that impinges on the system.

Person or client

A person is seen as an adaptive system: a biopsychosocial being in constant interaction with the changing environment. Two major mechanisms allow adaptation and coping: the regulator and the cognator. The regulator mechanism is concerned with neural, endocrine and perception/psychomotor processes of perception, and the cognator mechanism is concerned with the processes of perception, learning, judgement and emotion. In addition, each person has four subsystems: the physiologic, self-concept, role function and interdependence relations. Coping and adaptation use both innate and acquired mechanisms which are biologic, psychologic and social in origin (Roy 1980).

Environment

Roy (1980) describes the environment as including 'all conditions, circumstances and influences surrounding and affecting the development and behaviour of persons or groups' (p. 269).

Health

Health is seen as a state of being and becoming an integrated whole person; that is, the condition in which needs are met and integrity is maintained because of adaptation. A person's adaptation is a function of the stimuli he or she is exposed to and his or her adaptation level. Adaptation level is determined by the combined effect of three types of stimuli:

1. focal stimuli—the stimuli immediately confronting the person
2. contextual stimuli—all other stimuli present
3. residual stimuli—the beliefs, attitudes and traits of the person which have an indeterminate effect on the present situation.

Nursing

Nursing is the practice of facilitating the adaptation of an individual's four subsystems, or adaptive modes (the physiologic, self-concept, role function and interdependence relations). The nurse attempts to modify or maintain stimuli affecting adaptation within the nursing process. Nursing assessment focuses on two units of analysis: the person's system and environmental interaction, while intervention is concerned with manipulation of parts of the system or environment. Nursing assessment is conducted on two levels. Firstly, the nurse identifies client behaviours in each of the adaptive modes in order to situate the client's position on the health-illness continuum. Secondly, the nurse attempts to identify focal, contextual and residual factors influencing behaviours. The nursing diagnosis which follows is a statement of the relationship between behaviour and the impinging stimuli. Interventions consist of selecting the influencing factors which can be manipulated (Roy 1980).

The community

Roy's adaptation model provides a useful guide to community health nursing. As in the Neuman model, the community is conceptualized as a system. According to the adaptation model, the system or community has four subsystems or modes of care: the physiological, self-concept, role function and interdependence.

The physiological subsystem consists of the community's size, location, physical and geographical features and hazards, and its population. Community self-concept is reflected in such aspects as the degree of mobility or sense of permanence of its residents, and the degree of care taken to improve or preserve the community in its functional or adaptive state. Role function can be described in relation to intracommunity relationships; that is, the extent to which organizational and social roles within the community contribute to its adaptation level. Intercommunity and intracommunity relationships also reflect the community's role function and therefore its adaptation level. Interactions between all subsystems, and between the community and its wider social system indicate the level of adaptation within the interdependence mode.

Assessing the level of adaptation in all four modes constitutes the first stage of community assessment. The second stage involves an examination of the focal, contextual and residual stimuli influencing any areas of maladaptation. Focal stimuli include such things as health promoting characteristics (clean air, healthful climate) or health and safety hazards within the environment. Contextual stimuli include access to health care and availability of resources. Residual stimuli include those factors which constitute a social profile of the community; such as beliefs, attitudes, traits, propensity to utilize health services or to engage in self-care.

Nursing intervention is indicated when all stimuli lie outside the client's zone of adaptation (Clark 1984). In other words, the client does not have the capacity to deal with the problem without some type of outside intervention. The nurse then becomes an advocate for change. Nursing actions for primary prevention include heightening community awareness of the focal, contextual and residual stimuli in all four subsystems so that adaptive behaviours influenced by such stimuli can be encouraged and promoted. For example, in the case of an environmental pollutant, programs could be instituted which would monitor the pollutant and educate community inhabitants on the risk factors and alternative risk reduction behaviours associated with it. Secondary prevention would focus on the outcomes of maladaptive stimuli. Interventions would be aimed at modifying or eliminating the source of the pollution and, for those affected by the maladaptive condition, providing care or assisting with self-care. Tertiary prevention would aim at long term restorative planning to rehabilitate those affected by the pollutant and to advocate for alternatives (such as government policies) which would allow the community a more adaptive pollution free environment.

Self-care: Orem's self-care nursing model

Orem's model focuses primarily on interactionist and developmental perspectives. The model revolves around the concept of self-care, which refers to an adult's continuous contribution to his or her own continued existence, health and well being. The concept is extended to cover dependent self-care, such as an adult's contribution to the health and well being of dependent members of the social group, including children (Orem 1980).

Each individual has certain self-care requisites (needs). The ability to meet those requisites is called the self-care agency (ability) and depends upon such factors as age, general state of health, usual pattern of response to internal and external stimuli, values and goals, available resources and the extent of health care knowledge (Orem 1971). When the self-care agency is less than optimal, a self-care deficit is said to exist.

Person or client

Orem (1980) describes the person or client as one who is biologically, symbolically and socially functional.

Environment

Environment is mentioned in the self-care model as the context in which the nurse assists the client in developing an ability for self-care to meet present or future demands for action (Orem 1980).

Health

Health is a state of being whole and sound, linked to an individual's stage of growth and development. The physical, psychological, interpersonal and social aspects are inseparable, and relate to self-care requisites in three categories:

Universal self-care requisites—maintenance of a sufficient intake of air, water, food; provision of care associated with elimination processes and excrements; maintenance of a balance between solitude and social interaction; prevention of hazards to human life, functioning and well being; promotion of human functioning and development within social groups in accord with human potential, known human limitations and the human desire to be normal.

Developmental self-care requisites—the bringing about and maintenance of living conditions that support life processes and promote human progress toward higher organization and maturation; provision of care either to prevent the occurrence of deleterious effects of conditions that can affect human development or to mitigate or overcome these conditions.

Health deviation self-care requisites—those due to illness, injury, specific forms of pathology including defects and disabilities, medical diagnosis and treatment (Orem 1980).

Nursing

Orem (1980) describes nursing as a 'creative effort of one human being to help another human being' (p. 55). Nursing is a helping system which can be wholly compensatory; that is, the client is unable to achieve self-care, therefore has health deviation self-care requisites; partly compensatory where both nurse and client work to achieve self-care; or supportive-educative, where the client is able to perform, or can and should perform self-care but does not do so without assistance.

Nursing agency is the ability to act as a nurse. Its requisites are a nursing self-concept, knowledge, experience, mastery of the operations of nursing practice, a skill repertoire and sustaining motives which produce a willingness to provide nursing care (Orem 1980).

The community

The self-care model is appropriate to both the ideology and practice of community health nursing. As with the individual, a community's universal self-care requisites include healthy air, water, food and elimination systems, as well as having social and safety needs met. Developmental self-care requisites include such things as meeting the collective physical and social needs of a growing or diminishing population, and providing for the needs of its residents according to their developmental stage. This is reflected in the adequacy of employment, housing, schools and recreational facilities for young and middle-aged families, and residential and recreational facilities for the elderly. Health deviation self-care requisites relate to the need for such therapeutic facilities as medical care institutions, home care programs, availability of health care personnel, community liaison services and self-help groups.

Community self-empowerment can be thought of as the ultimate goal of nursing. At the primary level of prevention the nurse promotes self-care through the supportive-educative helping system. For example, the nurse may assess the community's nutritional needs and educate residents on ways to use local foodstuffs to ensure adequate nutrition. At the secondary level of prevention, inadequacies in the local food supply would be redressed. Treatment for nutritional deficiencies and assistance with securing supplemental nutrients would be an example of using either a wholly compensatory or partly compensatory helping system. At the tertiary level, the nurse combines supportive-educative and partly compensatory systems to collaborate with the community in planning for long term restoration and maintenance of local nutritional needs, thereby contributing to the community's self-care agency.

Health promotion: Pender's health promotion model

Pender (1987) describes her health promotion model as an organizational framework for theory development and research in the area of health promoting behaviour. The model is derived from social learning theory which emphasizes the importance of cognitive mediating processes in the regulation of behaviour. Structurally, it is organized similarly to the health belief model (see Fig. 3.3). The health belief model, widely used by medical sociologists, is based on the premise that one's beliefs about health and illness determine health behaviour (Becker 1974).

In Pender's model, determinants of health promoting behaviour are categorized into cognitive-perceptual factors (individual perceptions), modifying factors and variables affecting the likelihood of action. Cognitive-perceptual factors are identified within the model as motivational mechanisms: those perceptions which predispose an individual to engage in health promoting behaviours. Included are the individual's perceptions regarding the importance of health, control of health, self-efficacy, definition of health, health status, benefits of health promoting behaviour and barriers to health promoting behaviour (Pender 1987).

The cognitive-perceptual mechanisms are modified by:

- demographic characteristics (age, sex, race, ethnicity, education, income)
- biological characteristics (for example, body weight)
- interpersonal influences, which include the expectations of significant others, family patterns of health care, and interactions with health professionals
- situational factors such as the availability and ease of access to health promoting alternatives
- behavioural factors, which include previous experience with health promoting actions, and cognitive and psychomotor skills necessary to implement health promoting behaviours (Pender 1987).

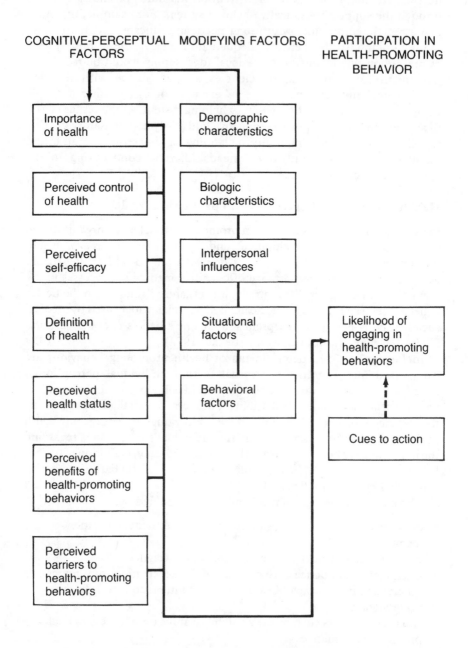

Fig. 3.3 Pender's health promotion model (From Pender 1987).

Other factors influencing health behaviours are cues to action, such as events which occur in the individual's environment. These activating cues interact with an individual's motivation to influence whether the individual will engage in health promoting behaviours (Rosenstock 1974, Pender 1987).

Person or client

The model takes a humanistic view of the individual, proposing that individuals have a basic striving or motivation for actualization as well as stability. Pender (1987) describes the actualizing tendency as 'the driving force toward increased levels of well being' (p. 9). As a complementary factor, the stabilizing tendency is responsible for 'protective manoeuvers', primarily maintaining a steady state of the internal and external environments. The expression of both actualizing and stabilizing tendencies is critical to integrated and healthy human functioning (Pender 1987).

Environment

According to Pender (1987), the environment includes the physical, interpersonal, and economic circumstances in which individuals reside.

Health

In Pender's (1987) view (referred to also in Ch. 1), health is 'the actualization of inherent and acquired human potential through goal-directed behaviour, competent self-care, and satisfying relationships with others while adjustments are made as needed to maintain structural integrity and harmony with the environment' (p. 27).

Nursing

Pender's model embraces a nursing role which focuses on comprehensive planning for health promotion and preventive care for individuals, families and communities. Health promotion includes those activities which encourage increasingly higher levels of well being and actualizing the health potential of individuals, families, communities and society. Prevention, or health protecting activities are aimed at helping the client avoid encumbrances throughout the life cycle that may prevent the emergence of optimum health (Pender 1987). The nurse functions as an agent of change, promoting health at the primary, secondary and tertiary levels (see Ch. 1).

Community health nurses have an ideal opportunity for health promotion and for serving as role models for healthy behaviours because of their recognized expertise and frequent, continuing contact with clients. Success in assisting individuals or groups to change personal health habits or health service use patterns depends upon an accurate understanding of cultural and personal perceptions, attitudes and values relevant to the target behaviours. As an initial step, the nurse must therefore make an accurate assessment of these perceptions, attitudes and values. Next, cues to action and motivational factors influencing behaviour must be examined. Intervention is then aimed at changing erroneous or unrealistic beliefs, cues or motivators in an attempt to elicit behaviour change. However, the nurse must also guard against blaming the victim, and work towards ensuring that the environment in which behaviour change is to occur is conducive to change, and will provide mechanisms whereby healthy behaviours can be supported.

The community

In Pender's model, a healthy community can be seen as one which combines actualization of its potential with stability and structural integrity. This is achieved through reciprocal interactions across support systems within and between communities, their environments and social systems. Community health promotion strategies must be targeted to the community's perceptions, modifying factors and variables affecting the likelihood of action. A community's perceptions of its health and health related needs will be a major determinant as to the likelihood of success of health promotion or illness prevention strategies.

For example, a suburban, white middle class community may be considered a healthy place to live, exhibit signs of pride in its citizens and surroundings, show visible indications through health and safety campaigns that health is valued, and take pride in its local autonomy through fund raising and community planning. Due to its receptiveness to health promotion practices, such a community could be considered a potential target for health promotion campaigns. However, if an AIDS prevention program were introduced, it may be that demographic variables (age, sex, race, ethnicity), interpersonal variables (relationship patterns) and situational variables (no reported cases of AIDS in the community) would modify the decision to accept or reject the program (the likelihood of action).

As an advocate for change, the nurse would attempt to shift the community's perceptions to a belief that the program and its outcome (prevention of the disease) was necessary for community actualization and stability. At the primary level of prevention, the nurse would seek to heighten awareness of the need for such a program by focusing educational messages on the modifying factors. This may include providing information on the incidence and prevalence of the disease across all demographic categories and identifying high risk behaviours rather than high risk groups. Once a shift in perceptions was evident, the nurse would then attempt to enhance the likelihood of the community conducting the program, by addressing any barriers to action (unavailable funds) and enhancing cues to action (supplementing a media campaign with a school information campaign).

Knowledge of the interpersonal factors modifying a community's perceptions of AIDS and AIDS victims can help to direct nursing efforts toward instituting self-help groups for those afflicted with the disease (secondary prevention). At the tertiary level, programs designed to maintain positive and supportive attitudes to those being treated for the disease become more appropriate when modifying factors (such as the presence or absence of community support groups), or cues to action (an epidemic in the community) are known.

Other models and theories

Taylor and McLaughlin (1991) explain that there are several nursing models which explore the articulation between community and the 'understandings of nursing' (p. 153). They cite three of McKay and Segall's (1983) four models which have an emphasis on the aggregate, or collective. These are the aggregate model, with nursing focused at the population level; the aggregate/administration model which is focused on the nursing unit or agency; and the aggregate family and group model, which emphasizes interacting social groups. Chalmers and Kristjanson (1989) also describe models with relevance to community health. Their models include the public health model, the community participation model, and the community change model. Hanchett (1990) reviewed nursing models in relation to the community as client, and concluded that the models of Orem (1980), Roy (1980), Smith (1983), and Rogers (1986) all contribute to the understanding of community health from a nursing perspective.

Stewart (1990) examined nursing models from a primary health care perspective and concluded that most conceptual models in nursing have only a superficial focus on the person-environment interaction. She suggests a community/environment/social support model to guide family and community health education and practice.

Parse's (1981, 1987) theory is one which has thus far been overlooked in the community health nursing literature. However, Rasmusson, Jonas and Mitchell (1991) used her theory to guide their efforts at counselling homeless youth. These authors found Parse's theory a refreshing change from those which revolve around problem solving. Parse (1981) suggests that human beings must be viewed as irreducible unities who achieve health by becoming true to oneself. Nursing practice revolves around enhancing the individual's quality of life, free of predetermined expectations. The theory proved useful to Rasmusson et al (1991) in guiding clinical practice; however, it presents an example of nursing individuals in the community rather than nursing the community. It is important to consider nursing models and theories from the perspective of utility. To be useful there must be a good fit between the theoretical propositions and the particular nursing goal(s), whether they relate to education, research or practice.

Family theories

Whall and Fawcett (1991) suggest that the nursing (meta) paradigm should be modified to account for family phenomena and to place family theory development within a nursing perspective. These authors advance the notion that there has been professional interest in the family as a unit of nursing care since Nightingale's time, and that family theory development is now a vital component of nursing's knowledge base.

Many of the traditional theorists mention the family in their discussion of the person/client (King 1981, Neuman 1982, Roy 1980, Orem 1985, Rogers 1990). However, there is today a growing number of theorists who are sensitized to the need for explicit family theories (e.g. Lobo, cited in Whall & Fawcett 1991). Many researchers have begun to contribute to family theory development by studying family phenomena ranging from the effects of sociopolitical forces on the family (Heistand 1982), to more specific issues such as the effect of pregnancy on the family system (Fawcett 1989), step-parenting (Stern 1982), family violence (Meister 1984), social support (Kane 1988, Frey 1989) and separated families (Hanson 1986, McMurray 1992). One of the most interesting and well developed theories has emerged from the work of Friedemann (1989a, 1989b) whose synthesis of earlier theories has provided a basis for her theory which relates to family mental health. It is anticipated that as more nurse theorists come to recognize the importance of the family in community health, the momentum for family theory development will increase.

SUMMARY

Conceptual models provide a useful tool to guide the practice of community health nursing. The models chosen for the previous discussion conceptualize the community as a system of interacting subsystems, as a basis for adaptation, as a situation for self-care and as a forum for health promotion in the family as well as the community at large. Regardless of the model used, the process of nursing remains constant. The community is assessed, issues are identified, interventions are planned, then executed at the primary, secondary and tertiary levels, and the entire process is evaluated to review its strengths and areas for improvement. The chapter to follow explores this process as it relates to the health problems and issues of communities.

Study exercises

---

1. Provide an example of how Pender's health promotion model can be used to help a community which is predominantly Aboriginal.
2. Provide an example of how Orem's model can be used for promoting sexual health in a group of adolescents.
3. Explain how a systems model could be used to guide behaviour change in a group of male executives who have come to a quit smoking class.
4. Describe how you would use Roy's adaptation model as a framework for health education in a farming community.
5. Choose a model which was not examined in this chapter and discuss its usefulness for helping victims of child sexual abuse.

REFERENCES

Aamodt A 1991 Ethnography and epistemology: generating nursing knowledge. In: Morse J (ed) Qualitative nursing research: a contemporary dialogue. Sage Publications, Newbury Park, pp 40-53

Becker M 1974 The health belief model and personal health behaviour. Slack, Thorofare

Benedict M, Behringer Sproles J 1982 Application of the Neuman model to public health nursing practice. In: Neuman B (ed) The Neuman systems model. Appleton-Century-Crofts, Norwalk, pp 223-237

Bertalanffy L 1952 Problems of life: an evaluation of modern biological and scientific thought. Harper & Row, New York

Chalmers K, Kristjanson L 1989 The theoretical basis for nursing at the community level: a comparison of three models. Journal of Advanced Nursing 14:569-574

Clark M 1984 Community nursing: health care for today and tomorrow. Reston Publishing, Reston

Fawcett J 1989 Spouses' experiences during pregnancy and the postpartum: a program of research and theory development. Image: Journal of Nursing Scholarship 21:149-152

Frey M 1989 Social support and health: a theoretical formulation derived from King's conceptual framework. Nursing Science Quarterly 2(3):138-148

Friedemann M 1989a Closing the gap between grand theory and mental health practice with families, Part 1: the framework of systemic organization for nursing of families and family members. Archives of Psychiatric Nursing 3:10-19

Friedemann M 1989b Closing the gap between grand theory and mental health practice with families, Part 2: the control-congruence model for mental health nursing of families. Archives of Psychiatric Nursing 3:20-28

Hanchett E 1990 Nursing models and community as client. Nursing Science Quarterly 3(2):67-72

Hanson S 1986 Healthy single parent families. Family Relations 35:125-132

Heistand W 1982 Nursing, the family, and the 'new' social history. Advances in Nursing Science 4(3):1-12

Kane C 1988 Family social support: toward a conceptual model. Advances in Nursing Science 10(2):18-25

Kenney J 1990 Relevance of theoretical approaches in nursing practice. In: Christenson P, Kenney J (eds) Nursing process: application of conceptual models, 3rd edn. C V Mosby, St Louis, pp 3-19

King I 1981 A theory for nursing: system, concepts process. Wiley, New York

Lee G, Lancaster J 1988 Conceptual models for community health nursing. In: Stanhope M, Lancaster J (eds) Community health nursing: process and practice for promoting health, 2nd edn. C V Mosby, St Louis, pp 131-148

McFarlane J 1986 The value of models for care. In: Kershaw B, Savage J (eds) Models for nursing. Wiley, Chichester, pp 1-6

McKay R 1986 Theories, models, and systems for nursing. In: Nicoll L (ed) Perspectives on nursing theory. Little Brown, Boston, pp 199-207

McKay R, Segall M 1983 Methods and models for the aggregate. Nursing Outlook 31:328-334

McMurray A 1992 Influences on parent-child relationships in non-custodial mothers. Australian Journal of Marriage & Family 13(3):137-147

Meister S 1984 Family well being. In: Campbell J, Humphreys J (eds) Nursing care of victims of family violence. Reston Publishing, Reston, pp 53-73

Meleis A 1985 Theoretical nursing: development and process. J B Lippincott, Philadelphia

Neuman B 1982 The Neuman systems model. Appleton-Century-Crofts, Norwalk

Neuman B 1989 The Neuman systems model, 2nd edn. Appleton-Lange, Norwalk

Orem D 1971 Nursing: concepts of practice. McGraw-Hill, New York

Orem D 1980 Nursing: concepts of practice, 2nd edn. McGraw-Hill, New York

Orem D 1985 Nursing: concepts of practice, 3rd edn. McGraw-Hill, New York

Parse R 1981 Man-living-health: a theory of nursing. Wiley, New York

Parse R 1987 Nursing science: major paradigms, theories and critiques, W B Saunders, Philadelphia

Pender N 1987 Health promotion in nursing practice, 2nd edn. Appleton & Lange, Norwalk

Rapaport A 1968 Foreword. In: Buckley W (ed) Modern systems research for the behavioural scientist. Aldine, Chicago

Rasmusson D, Jonas C, Mitchell G 1991 The eye of the beholder: Parse's theory with homeless individuals. Clinical Nurse Specialist 5(3):139-143

Reed K 1989 Family theory related to the Neuman Systems Model. In: Neuman B (ed) The Neuman systems model, 2nd edn. Appleton & Lange, Norwalk, pp 385-395

Reed K 1993 Adapting the Neuman systems model for family nursing. Nursing Science Quarterly 6(2):93-97

Rogers M 1986 Science of unitary human beings. In: Malinsky M (ed) Exploration of Martha Rogers' science of unitary human beings, Appleton-Century-Crofts, Norwalk, pp 3-8

Rogers M 1990 Nursing: science of unitary, irreducible, human beings: update 1990. In: Barrett E (ed) Visions of Rogers' science-based nursing. National League for Nursing, New York, pp 5-11

Rosenstock I 1974 Historical origins of the health belief model. In: Becker M (ed) The health belief model and personal health behaviour. Slack, Thorofare, pp 1-8

Roy C 1980 The Roy adaptation model. In: Riehl J, Roy C (eds) Conceptual models for nursing practice, 2nd edn. Appleton-Century-Crofts, New York, pp 179-188

Smith J 1983 The idea of health. Teachers College Press, New York

Stern P 1982 Affiliating in stepfather families: teachable strategies leading to stepfather-child friendship. Western Journal of Nursing Research 4:75-89

Stewart M 1990 From provider to partner: a conceptual framework for nursing education based on primary health care premises. Advances in Nursing Science 12(2):9-27

Taylor S, McLaughlin K 1991 Orem's general theory of nursing and community nursing. Nursing Science Quarterly 4(4):153-160

Whall A, Fawcett J 1991 Family theory development in nursing: state of the science and art. F A Davis, Philadelphia

Yura H, Walsh M 1967 The nursing process: assessing, planning, implementing, evaluating. Appleton-Century-Crofts, New York

4. The process of nursing in the community

In order to link the theoretical foundations of nursing to practice activities, some examination of the *process* of nursing is necessary. The theorists mentioned in the previous chapter contend that a healthy community is one in which most members' needs are met and there is a state of balance between the forces maintaining stability and those which energize the community. Some of these forces are beyond the control of either the nurse or community residents. However, the community health nurse can function in partnership with the community to assist and enable its members to meet community needs through systematic and thoughtful planning.

Planning is a bilateral process in the community in that priorities must be set according to both client need and the goals of the organization which usually reflect global, national and local health priorities. For example, the school nurse who establishes a nutrition awareness program in the school demonstrates a commitment to organizational and national public health goals for improving the community's nutritional status. To achieve a balance between meeting individual client needs and promoting the health of the entire community requires strong organizational skills. These skills can be developed and refined by using a 'process-oriented' approach to practice in which the intellectual, interpersonal and technical skills of nursing practice can be systematized (Kenney 1991).

THE NURSING PROCESS

The *nursing process*, originally devised by Yura and Walsh (1967), is familiar to most nurses as a framework for planning nursing care. It is a five-stage process which consists of assessment, diagnosis, planning, implementation and evaluation (Alfaro 1986). Initially, needs are assessed, then analyzed in order to identify a nursing diagnosis. Nursing intervention is planned according to what the nurse judges to be the individual's, family's or community's priorities, then the plan is implemented and evaluated. The process is systematic, yet adaptable to different client populations and situations. It is a logical yet circular process in which ongoing evaluation of each step can result in activity being directed to any of the previous steps to monitor the usefulness of decisions and plans. For those who accept

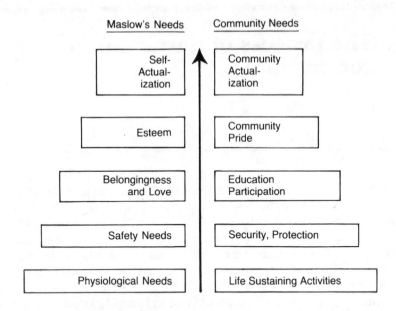

Fig. 4.1 A comparison of Maslow's identification of basic needs of the individual with those of the community as client (From Higgs & Gustafson 1985).

Maslow's theory that needs can be hierarchically structured from the most to the least vital, the needs of a community can be configured into a structure which parallels Maslow's hierarchy of individual needs (see Fig. 4.1). This type of prioritization is based on the premise that lower level needs must be met before the higher level needs can be realized.

Although the nursing process has been widely accepted by nurses in a variety of settings throughout the past three decades, it is somewhat oversimplified for community health nursing. A study of the practice activities of expert community health nurses conducted by the author revealed that the process of nursing in the community revolves around two main goals: self-management and client management. As illustrated in Figure 4.2, self-management consists of planning the case load or clinic, organizing for personal needs such as time, space, transportation and information, and forward planning for such matters as educational needs. Client management begins when the nurse establishes contact and rapport, and involves an investigative process of screening and interviewing. During client assessment interviews, cues emerge which form the basis of clinical judgements. The judgement process consists of attending to these cues, judging the situation, validating judgements with the client, and setting priorities for meeting the needs of the client. The nurse's involvement in enabling needs to be met consists of one or more of the following activities: advising, reassuring, explaining, counselling, and referring. Finally, the nurse engages in a variety of activities aimed at monitoring progress. These activities are accompanied by meticulous documentation and include ongoing surveillance, co-ordination activities related to client needs, and evaluating outcomes (McMurray 1992).

This model of community health nursing practice represents an extension of the traditional nursing process. In preparation for meeting client needs, the nurse assesses her or his own needs related to time, space, transportation and information as a basis for planning the day's (or the week's) activities. In the context of client management, self-management needs for both the immediate and long term may be reviewed and revised as necessary. For example, the nurse may encounter a unique and unfamiliar problem and

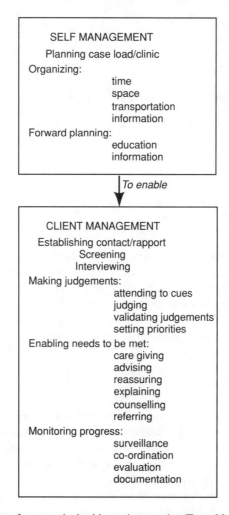

Fig. 4.2 The process of community health nursing practice (From McMurray 1992).

CLIENT MANAGEMENT

Assessment ———— Establishing contact/rapport
　data gathering ———— Screening
　analysis ———— Interviewing
　　　　Making judgements:
　　　　　　　　attending to cues
Diagnosis ———— judging
　　　　　　　　validating judgements
Planning ———— setting priorities
Implementation — Enabling needs to be met:
　　　　　　　care giving
　　　　　　　advising
　　　　　　　reassuring
　　　　　　　explaining
　　　　　　　counselling
　　　　　　　referring
Evaluation ———— Monitoring progress:
　　　　　　　surveillance
　　　　　　　co-ordination
　　　　　　　evaluation
　　　　　　　documentation

Fig. 4.3 The process of client management within the context of the nursing process (From McMurray 1992).

decide to seek further information by reading, studying, researching and/or networking with colleagues. In this way, the nurse moves back and forth between self-management and client management activities so that the process remains cyclical rather than sequential.

As Figure 4.3 illustrates, the process of client management can be seen within the context of the traditional nursing process.

THE NURSING PROCESS IN COMMUNITY HEALTH NURSING PRACTICE

The nursing process involves a deliberate series of actions directed towards an outcome. The outcome of nursing activities in the community may be that a family develops new ways to improve the health of its members, or that certain members of the community have greater access to health services, or that an illness or epidemic is prevented by immunization, or all of these things. Systematizing the process and employing common conventions for documenting care are aimed at ensuring that as many community needs as possible are met, either by direct intervention, referral to appropriate resources, or self-care.

Assessment

Data gathering

The initial stage of the nursing process consists of data gathering. Although the content varies somewhat, the skills and strategies used to assess a community are similar to those used in assessing an individual or family. The first step consists of observing the general appearance of all physical elements of the community, then deciding what needs to be assessed in greater detail. Ideally, assessment data is a combination of this observational data with interview and survey information, but the amount of information obtained will depend upon what information is available, the nurse's time and resources, and the willingness and disposition of the community towards participating in the data gathering process, all of which point to the need for developing contact and rapport with key members of the community.

The views of formal and informal opinion leaders and a cross-section of community residents often provides a helpful sample of community attitudes and beliefs, as well as an historical perspective of current issues and concerns. Interviews should be open-ended, but directed, planned and organized in order to provide objective information on the community's needs, motives and conflicts (Fromer 1979). A community forum approach may also be taken, wherein residents are invited to express their concerns at a public meeting, as long as community interviews and observations are also conducted. Although the 'town hall' approach may bring many residents together at one time, often the opinions presented are those of the vocal articulate few, rather than the private majority.

Community surveys and previous screening reports are another source of valuable information. Health departments, libraries and universities often have epidemiological information on the occurrence and distribution of health disorders in the population. Telephone books, city directories, newspapers and community agencies also provide survey information on community resources, sociomedical indicators and environmental indices. Once these resources have been tapped, the information can be categorized to provide a clear picture of the community's health status.

Organization of data

A thorough assessment should be guided by a framework which addresses the physical and social aspects of the community. The community assessment tool devised by Clark (1984) presents a well organized, comprehensive guide to data gathering (see Appendix 2). Categories of information include the following:

1. General description of the community. Included in this category are the location, physical geography or topology of a community and its climate; the size, density and type of community (rural or urban); the community's history; its political structure and distribution of power; and its patterns of population change.

2. *Population characteristics.* Characteristics of the community's population include age, sex, race and language, income level, education, religion, employment patterns, marital status and family composition.

3. *Environmental factors.* These factors include housing, water supply and waste disposal, protective services, accessibility of transportation, availability of educational facilities, communication systems, recreation and nuisance factors.

4. *Health status indicators.* Indicators of a community's health status can be of two types: biostatistics, that is, the vital statistics of birth rates, morbidity and mortality rates; and health promotion indicators, such as immunization levels and general nutritional status, existence of health education and health promotion programs in the community, availability and utilization of preventive health services.

5. *Attitudes toward health.* A community's attitudes toward health are reflected in its definition of health and illness, and the relative value placed on wellness, as evidenced by local government budget allocations and spending patterns for health care.

6. *Community relationships with society.* Within this category is information on the relative autonomy of the community to provide goods and services, the free flow of ideas and goods, and the factors either facilitating this flow or those which indicate social isolation.

Cultural assessment

As mentioned in Chapter 1, needs are influenced by such factors as class, culture, gender, age, language, values, education and economic reality (Lawler 1991). Thus theories such as Maslow's (1943), which suggest a predetermined sequence of needs, have yet to be proven generalizeable to all types of communities. For this reason, the initial stage of the nursing process must also include cultural assessment, particularly in multicultural communities. Assessment of the basic cultural needs of community groups includes ethnic affiliation, religious preference, family patterns, food patterns, and ethnic health care practices. This information will give sufficient information to determine if further, indepth assessment of cultural factors is needed (Tripp-Reimer, Brink & Saunders 1984). These authors suggest that cultural assessment must be reflexive; that is, it must include information on how the client group perceives the group or community's values, customs and beliefs and how they wish to fit in within the normative patterns.

Analysis

This second stage of community assessment involves attending to the cues which arise from the assessment data in order to analyze and interpret the information. This analysis and interpretation forms the basis for clinical judgements or nursing diagnoses. Analysis of the data should yield a community profile from which the nurse attempts to identify community strengths, major community problems and/or health issues, and current or proposed community actions for problem resolution (Burgess 1983). Clark (1984) suggests that several questions need to be asked at this stage, such as:

- What is going on physically or socially and how is it manifest?
- What are the givens? (history, constraints, facilitating factors)
- What feelings, perceptions or attitudes are being expressed or experienced?
- What appears to be unusual, unexpected or atypical?
- What has changed and how is the community coping?
- What is the best-case scenario? (favourable outcome)
- What is the worst-case scenario? (unfavourable outcome)

Nursing diagnosis

The nursing diagnosis is a tentative statement or hypothesis regarding a health problem or issue which is amenable to nursing intervention (Clark 1984, Higgs & Gustafson 1985). It is a tentative judgement in that it is based on initial assessment and will be updated and completed following further data collection and validation with the community. Generating the nursing diagnosis represents a critical stage in the nursing process as it epitomizes the process of making clinical judgements. The nursing diagnosis should describe health concerns, strengths and resources, and imply an aetiology (Anderson & McFarlane 1988, Kenney 1991). It should be written in the format of a problem-oriented record, with the initial description, identification of factors aetiologically related to the problem, and the signs and symptoms of the problem.

Each nursing diagnosis should be validated by both *subjective* and *objective* information. A summary *assessment* is then made, and tentative *plans* or strategies suggested. The SOAP (Subjective, Objective, Assessment, Plan) format is a helpful guide to use in documenting this stage. Subjective data represent information which is reported by community members and indicates the way in which people *experience* a problem. Objective data are derived from the nurse's *observations* and from defined sources of health status information such as epidemiological studies and/or hospital, health agency or community service reports. The assessment statement represents the nurse's judgement of the situation and health needs and the plan summarizes the initial approach which the nurse has decided to adopt to deal with the issues and needs in order of priority. Some examples follow.

Example 4.1: Community nutritional deficiencies: diagnosis

Inability to provide for the nutritional needs of community residents (initial description) related to a lack of arable land and isolation from other crop-producing communities (aetiological conditions) as evidenced by high incidence and prevalence of illness related to vitamin deficiencies (signs and symptoms).

Example 4.1.1: Community nutritional deficiencies: assessment and plan

Nursing diagnosis: Inability to provide for the nutritional needs of community residents related to the lack of arable land, and isolation from other crop-producing communities, as evidenced by a high incidence and prevalence of illness related to vitamin deficiencies.

Subjective: Community residents report that it is impossible to grow crops on their land and that the supply of fresh vegetables from elsewhere is sporadic.

Objective: Many members of the community appear thin and pale. Roads are impassable for five months of each year due to heavy rains. Hospital admissions for infections and nutritional deficiencies have increased by 8% annually for the past five years.

Assessment: The community requires a steady source of fresh food.

Plan:

- Approach community residents to gather any suggestions for solving the problem and to determine the history of any previous strategies used.
- Contact any other health professionals involved with the community to investigate possible collaborative strategies.
- Investigate possible neighbouring sources of food, and the costs of transporting it to the community by means other than land transport.
- Assess the community's financial resources and possible sources of food subsidies.
- Assist the community members to organize themselves to apply for funding or to petition the local government for assistance in overcoming the problem.

Example 4.2: Inadequate community safety: diagnosis

Difficulty in providing for the safety needs of community residents (initial description) related to large numbers of marauding youths and inadequate police surveillance (aetiological conditions) as evidenced by a high incidence of vandalism and resultant fearfulness of residents (signs and symptoms).

**Example 4.2.1: Inadequate community safety:
assessment and plan**

Nursing diagnosis: Difficulty in providing for the safety needs of community residents related to large numbers of marauding youths and inadequate police surveillance, as evidenced by a high incidence of vandalism and resultant fearfulness of residents.

Subjective: Community residents report that they fear leaving their homes because of a recent spate of broken windows, theft and muggings in the neighbourhood.

Objective: Attendance at community events has declined. Police statistics report theft and muggings have increased by 10% over last year. Police budgetary restrictions have resulted in halving the frequency of patrols to the community.

Assessment: A hazard to the safety of community residents exists.

Plan:

- Meet with community residents to clarify and itemize the incidence and types of crimes occurring.
- Contact any other health professionals involved with the community to investigate possible collaborative strategies.
- Suggest that a resident committee be formed to assist the police in safeguarding the community.
- Meet with the residents' committee to gather suggestions for a neighbourhood watch program, and a program of community education on safety and protection.
- Solicit guidance from the police or local government officials on ways in which they believe the problem might be overcome.

Example 4.3: Social isolation of the community's elderly: diagnosis

Social isolation of the community's elderly population (initial description) related to a lack of community and home health care (aetiological factors) as evidenced by a high rate of institutionalization of the frail elderly for extended periods of time (signs and symptoms).

Example 4.3.1: Social isolation of the community's elderly: assessment and plan

Nursing diagnosis: Social isolation of the community's elderly population related to a lack of community and home health care, as evidenced by a high rate of institutionalization of the frail elderly for extended periods of time.

Subjective: Families of the elderly report that they are unable to obtain adequate services to maintain ageing family members at home.

Objective: Hospital statistics indicate a high frequency of extended admissions for the frail elderly. No day care centres for the elderly exist in the community. Home care services have been decreased due to recent budget cuts, and the services of neighbouring communities are overburdened meeting local obligations.

Assessment: A need exists for community and home health care for the elderly.

Plan:

- Interview the hospitalized elderly to ask their opinions on existing and potential needs and services.
- Survey the families of the community to assess specific needs and potential utilization of services.
- Contact any other health professionals involved with the community to investigate possible collaborative strategies.
- Compile a list of medical conditions of the elderly which are currently being treated in hospital, which would be amenable to home or community care.
- Investigate possible sources of funding for day care nutrition and transportation services for the elderly.
- Explore existing community resources and services which could be expanded or adapted to fill the community's needs.

These examples illustrate how the nursing process is used when the community is the client. When the client is a family, a similar format is adopted.

Example 4.4: Parenting difficulties: diagnosis

Potential threat to family stability related to parents' lack of knowledge regarding parenting practices, as evidenced by discordant role relationship in the marital, parental and sibling subsystems.

Example 4.4.1: Parenting difficulties: assessment and plan

Nursing diagnosis: Potential threat to family stability related to parents' lack of knowledge regarding parenting practices, as evidenced by discordant role relationship in the marital, parental and sibling subsystems.

Subjective: Mother states that the children are always fighting, that she 'can't control them', and that her husband no longer comes home until they are in bed for the night.

Objective: Mother appears pale and drawn. Children (aged 2 and 4) compete for toys, pushing, screaming and biting. Neither child pays attention to mother's warnings or occasional slaps on the backside.

Assessment: The family would benefit from a less chaotic environment in which children are taught consistent behavioural guidelines, mother receives guidance in disciplining children and occasional respite from family responsibilities, and father participates in parenting and provides emotional support for his wife.

Plan:

- Explore the mother's knowledge and understanding of parenting practices in order to devise appropriate teaching strategies.
- Provide the family with information on child development and parenting skills, or refer them (if appropriate) to a parenting course.
- Assist the mother in exploring ways in which she and her husband could devise strategies for mutual support during this and other child rearing stages.
- Discuss the possibility of including the family's support network (extended family, friends) in planning to meet the family's goals.
- Encourage the mother to discuss her feelings on parenting and the marital relationship.
- Suggest local resources available to her for support and assistance, such as the community health centre, parent group, children's play group or women's self-help group.
- Discuss the idea of contracting with the mother to work on small changes in her approach to disciplining the children.
- Provide ongoing encouragement, support, guidance and follow-up for the family.

Documenting the information related to each problem or issue in such detail allows the nurse to look at the scope of the problem, and the potential commitment required for intervention. Under normal circumstances, it is difficult to accomplish all aspects of each plan within the typical time constraints, as most nurses are usually dealing with multiple issues and problems at any given time. However, decisions must be made as to the urgency and priority of each, and a condensed plan devised.

Planning

The planning phase of the nursing process is aimed at setting priorities, formulating goals and objectives in terms of expected outcomes, identifying available resources and constraints, developing collaborative and role modelling strategies, and choosing the apparently best solution to the problems or issues.

As mentioned previously, effective management of nursing care involves planning for both self and client needs. Planning may therefore involve techniques for time management. Turla and Hawkins (1983) suggest that one way of doing this is to use a priority-payoff grid (see Fig. 4.4). Here's how it works. At the beginning of the day, or at the end of the previous day, each activity is assigned to a box in the grid. Across the horizontal the boxes represent high, moderate or low priority. Down the vertical, they represent high, moderate or low payoff.

Going through the exercise of identifying activities by priority and payoff helps to clarify what the day (week or month) has in store. Once activities are designated to a certain box, time can be allocated to high priority, high payoff tasks first; while low priority, low payoff tasks can be left until later. For example, a home visit which must be made to a family with a diabetic member who is having problems controlling insulin dosage would be considered a high priority, high payoff case in relation to a routine follow-up visit for another family.

Even when the day is organized around a priority-payoff grid, it is important to build in time for unexpected events. One rule of thumb is to allocate times to the day's requirements, then build in an extra 15 minutes per hour for interruptions, phone calls and emergencies. Some days this is not enough, some days it is too much, but when averaged over the week or the month, 15 minutes per working hour is pretty typical of the 'interruption factor'.

One suggestion for setting priorities involves classifying problems according to the hierarchy of community needs shown in Figure 4.1. Those needs which are lower on the hierarchy receive higher priority than those higher up, so that lower level needs can be met before higher level needs. If all three of our hypothetical community examples (Examples 4.1, 4.2, 4.3) existed in the same community, the need for food (a life sustaining need) would be

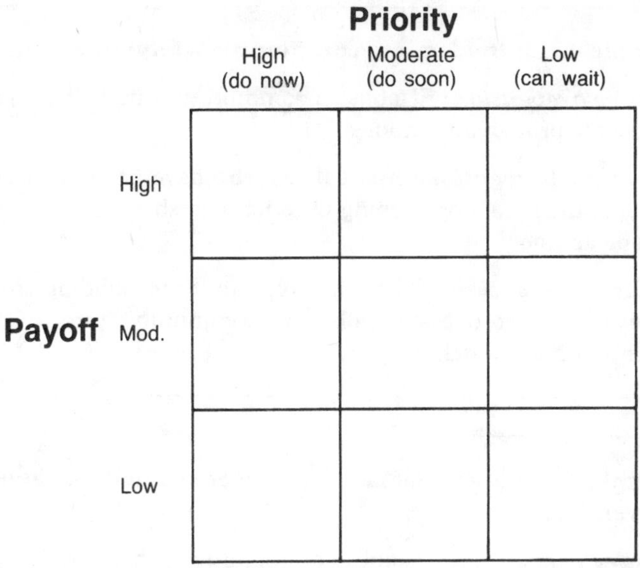

Priority

	High (do now)	Moderate (do soon)	Low (can wait)
High			
Mod.			
Low			

Payoff

Fig. 4.4 Priority payoff grid.

addressed first. Next, the need for safety would be attended to, and finally, the social isolation need.

Depending upon resources and the scope of the problem, the nursing plan may be aimed at any one or all of primary, secondary and tertiary levels of prevention and include care giving, advising, reassuring, explaining, counselling and referring (see Fig. 4.3). Referring to our previous examples, a plan for primary, secondary and tertiary prevention may be somewhat like the following:

Example 4.1.2: Community nutritional deficiencies: intervention

Primary prevention: Develop a program to educate community members on nutritional requirements and alternative sources of vitamins.

Secondary prevention: Provide care for those suffering from nutritional deficiencies.

Tertiary prevention: Assist the community in monitoring the progress of residents being rehabilitated from nutritionally related illness, and in devising a long term strategy for securing adequate food based on realistic resources and constraints.

Example 4.2.2: Inadequate community safety: intervention

Primary prevention: Establish a community education program to help people protect their homes.

Secondary prevention: Assist those who have been vandalized to overcome their fears by keeping in touch and sharing their concerns with one another.

Tertiary prevention: Assist the community in building trust and security through co-operative police and community efforts to establish a neighbourhood watch program.

Example 4.3.2: Social isolation of the community's elderly: intervention

Primary prevention: Establish a program which would inform the community and its funding agencies of the health advantages of community care for the frail elderly.

Secondary prevention: Attempt to arrange visits to the institutionalized and isolated elderly by community volunteers who would keep them in touch with one another and with events in the community.

Tertiary prevention: Assist the community in developing a long term strategy for including and reintegrating the elderly into the social environment of the community.

Example 4.4.2: Parenting difficulties: intervention

Primary prevention: Develop or refer the family to an educational program on positive parenting practices.

Secondary prevention: Provide counselling and support for the family.

Tertiary prevention: Monitor the family's progress, providing support and guidance.

To prepare for evaluating the effectiveness of the planning stage, plans can now be summarized into specific expected outcomes. Expected outcomes are guided by the acronym RUMBA. That is, they should be:

Realistic
Unambiguous
Measurable
Behavioural
Achievable.

For our examples, expected outcomes would be:

**Example 4.1.3: Community nutritional deficiencies:
expected outcome for primary prevention**

By the end of the year, a program to educate the community on nutrition will be conducted. It will take the form of a six session teaching program run in the school and include a nutrition poster competition for students, distribution of nutrition pamphlets to all new parents, and the launching of a newspaper column on nutrition jointly authored by the community health nurse and the regional nutrition consultant.

**Example 4.2.3: Inadequate community safety:
expected outcome for secondary prevention**

By the end of July, a 'neighbour to neighbour' support group will be established to initiate a system of making nightly reassuring telephone calls to all community residents who live alone.

**Example 4.3.3: Social isolation of the community's elderly:
expected outcome for tertiary prevention**

By the beginning of the new year, the community health team will submit a proposal to the state (or provincial) government to fund a program of community services to help the elderly recover from illness at home unless severely disabled. The program will consist of housekeeping, meals, transportation and health care services.

It is important to note that nursing interventions do not proceed sequentially from primary, to secondary, to tertiary prevention. In the process of prioritizing, the nurse needs to take into account the urgency of the situation, using the priority-payoff grid if necessary. In the example of the family experiencing parenting difficulties, an initial priority would be to secure temporary respite for the mother, then to proceed with guidance and teaching once she is more relaxed and receptive to new ideas. The first expected outcome would therefore be related to secondary prevention.

**Example 4.4.3: Parenting difficulties:
expected outcome for secondary prevention**

By next week's visit, mother will have taken one afternoon off from caretaking and engaged in a personally pleasurable activity. Following next week's visit, a new expected outcome may be set.

**Example 4.4.3: Parenting difficulties:
revised expected outcome for secondary prevention**

By next week's visit, mother will have read the information provided, and be prepared to discuss ideas and issues arising from the material.

This second expected outcome attempts to set the stage for primary prevention. Once the mother is ready, the nurse may seize upon the teachable moment, and provide health education and support. Together the mother and nurse will evaluate and revise expected outcomes throughout the course of the visits, to the point where there has been mutually satisfactory progress.

RUMBA?

All of the expected outcomes listed above have a defined time frame. All are presumably realistic and affordable in a developed country. The outcomes are stated concisely. Each is measurable in terms of what is to be accomplished. Each specifies behaviours which are to be undertaken, and appears to be achievable in the projected time. Unless unforeseeable circumstances impinge on the plans, the interventions should be successful.

Implementation

The successful implementation of a nursing plan depends upon skilful assessment which, in turn, depends upon mutual goal setting and ongoing communication between the nurse and the community or family. Assessment data may indicate relatively straightforward nursing actions or involve program development. When new programs or important changes are instituted, a community or a family goes through three major stages: unfreezing, moving and refreezing (Lewin 1958).

At the stage of unfreezing, the need for change is identified. At the moving stage, the community acknowledges the problems and the presence of a change agent, and various alternative solutions are considered. For example, when a new program is planned, several issues must be considered:

- securing strong leadership
- investigating legal authority and enforceable sanctions
- exploring financial arrangements
- obtaining the co-operation of private and public sectors
- securing support from those groups concerned with environmental and cultural issues
- involving those who will implement the program
- obtaining assistance from experts and specialists who can contribute to understanding the problem or issues and possible solutions
- maintaining the focus on health, rather than the program (Clark 1984, Anderson & McFarlane 1988).

Addressing these issues helps to identify the driving or restraining forces existing in the community. The third stage of change, refreezing, is described by Lewin (1958) as implementation of the program and stabilization of the situation. Actions aimed at maintaining stability will vary according to each situation and can be facilitated by continuing dialogue with those affected by the change.

Throughout the implementation process, communication is the most important variable. Plans, progress and new developments must be discussed among members of the community-care giver partnership, including other health care professionals regardless of whether the plan is directed towards the community, family or individual. Collaboration between members of the health care team and other agencies and resources is often the critical factor predicting success.

Resources

A resource, as defined by Clemen et al (1987), is 'an agency, group or individual that assists a client in meeting a need' (p. 292). Health care resources can be formal, that is, their primary purpose is the provision of health care services; or informal, in that they provide health care services but not as a primary function (Clemen et al 1987). Informal resources include relatives, self-help groups, and service organizations such as Rotary or Apex clubs which often raise funds for health care causes as only one of their activities in the community.

Most communities have available a directory of community resources and services. These are helpful for familiarizing oneself with the community and for making client referrals. Most nurses, however, find it necessary to compile their own directory, supplementing the local one with resources either familiar to them or recommended by colleagues. A typical directory lists emergency services, local physicians and other health care professionals, specialist services, government services, voluntary agencies, and professional networks. The list may be compiled from the telephone Yellow Pages, newspaper advertisements of community services, information circulars from local or national agencies, colleagues, and the employing agency or department. Each community's directory provides a unique window to the services and resources to be found there. Figure 4.5 lists typical directory headings.

The resource directory can be a loose-leaf book, a set of cards or a database compiled for computer storage. Clemen et al (1987) suggest the following information be displayed for each resource:

• Name of the resource—including address, phone number, name and title of the person in charge
• Purpose of services—such as financial aid to families, meal planning, transportation for people with disabilities
• Eligibility criteria—such as income level, degree of impairment etc.
• Application procedure—such as the necessity of a written referral or support documents from a physician, or whether a processing time delay usually occurs
• Fees—user fees, or insurance reimbursement procedures.
• Office hours and days available
• Geographic area served.

For each resource, a note should be made on what specific information that resource requires of its clients. Usually, the resource will request the client's name, address and telephone number, age, sex and marital status; the names and birth dates of family members and others living in the household; the medical care source and health history; financial status and records; a list of other resources with whom the client is presently working; and the reason for seeking referral (Clemen et al 1987).

Referral

Knowing what information will be requested helps the nurse to prepare for referring clients to a resource, and also helps to ensure that the client will have an accurate expectation of the information required in the referral process. The nurse should obtain written consent from the client to reveal this information, and should give the client an explanation of the extent to which particular information is to be shared.

When a referral is made, the nurse should make every effort to ensure that the client is ready to deal with the problem and knows what to expect from the resource. This is important in such referrals as family counselling, where clients may see the referral as a quick solution to a problem without realizing that it may be an extended process to which all family members must contribute. Once these issues have been discussed, the nurse and client(s)

Emergency Numbers:	Police
	Fire
	Ambulance
	Poison Control
Hotlines:	Health Info
	Specific Hotlines (AIDS, Aged, Others)
Physicians:	
Other Health Professionals:	
Specialist Services:	Disease Related (Diabetes, Arthritis)
	Age/Stage Specific (Child health)
	Women's Health, Refuge, Crisis Centre)
	Family Services
	Self-Help Services
Government Services:	Health Education/Promotion
	Health Agencies/Departments
	Social Services/Welfare
	Occupational Health, Safety
	Environmental Agencies
	Employment, Labour Relations
	Housing
	Financial Aid
	Legal Aid
	Community Action
Voluntary Services:	Non-Government Agencies
	Religious Servies (Pastoral Care,
	Salvation Army)
Professional:	Nursing Association, Interest Groups
	Union
	Nursing Networks
	Research Agencies
	Libraries, Bookshops
	Schools of Nursing

Fig. 4.5 Typical components of a community directory.

can establish mutually agreed upon goals for the referral and a strategy for evaluating the service provided (Clemen et al 1987).

The decision to refer

One of the most difficult challenges for the novice nurse is knowing when to refer a client to a more appropriate or extended service. Although there is no rule of thumb, a referral is usually made for the following reasons: when it is ethically correct, that is, when a situation is clearly beyond the nurse's competency level; when a client requests it; when the nurse could possibly manage the situation, but there is someone available better equipped to deal with it; or when there is no available back-up for what may be incomplete or inadequate care. Making a referral is a systematic, judging, and decision making process as the example to follow illustrates.

Example 4.5: To refer or not

The nurse practising in a rural community is called by a neighbour to come immediately to one of the local family farms. Arriving at the farm she sees the father of the household on the roof, yelling at the bank manager below (who was about to foreclose on his mortgage) that he is going to jump. The farmer's wife is pleading with him, while the children are running around in circles screaming at the bank manager, who is trying to placate the man. Clearly, the family is in chaos, and the nurse is the first on the scene, although the local police are not far away. What does she do?

In this situation, the isolated circumstances dictate that she must do what she can to manage the crisis without precipitating a worst case scenario (the farmer's suicide) or further upsetting the family. Plans for long term helping must be secondary to the initial management. Her first instinct is to remove the bank manager whose presence is provoking the situation. She calmly, but firmly, asks him to leave immediately, despite the fact that he is desperately trying to smooth over a bad situation. Next, she attempts to get the other family members to go inside in order to create a calmer climate for talking to the man. Finally, she begins to talk the man down from the roof, drawing upon the relationship of mutual respect which she has previously established with him and his family in the hope that it will provide a basis for rational discussion.

Once the man has calmed down and descended, the nurse suggests that he join his family inside so that they can have a few quiet moments together. She explains that she will stay for a while and help them to ease up from the situation, then return in the morning to see whether she can be of any assistance to them. Her plans are already being formulated, and primarily involve reassurance and counselling until the visiting family psychologist returns to the community next month. She tempers her plans to help with the knowledge that, as a member of a small community, she must try to intervene without invading the family's privacy in such things as financial matters.

In this case, there is no one to accept an immediate referral except the police, and they were not present at the time the family was in crisis. The next day she will try to set the stage for the family to explore various options, advising them to seek counselling when it is available. She will then investigate whether there is any social action which the community can take to ride through the difficult financial times. In a multi-serviced metropolitan area, this case would be referred on to social workers and/or family counsellors. However, in a more isolated environment, referrals are often not possible and case management involves interventions which draw upon the nurse's own knowledge, skills, intuition and, as mentioned in Chapter 2, the 'gift of the gab and guts'!

Evaluation

One of the most important steps in the process of nursing is to monitor client progress toward meeting the expected outcomes of nursing care plans. This is accomplished through evaluative strategies which include surveillance, primarily through observing and assessing community members' changing health status, co-ordination of community services and support, evaluating the merit of nursing interventions and careful documentation of all stages of the process.

It is occasionally the case that a course of action or program for implementing a nursing plan ceases to be health promoting, yet is continued by over-zealous advocates who have invested much time and energy into its development. In these cases, both formative and summative evaluation provide the basis for deciding whether to terminate a plan or shift strategies. Ongoing, or formative evaluation measures progress towards goals and objectives, while summative evaluation measures outcomes. Evaluation questions which must be asked include:

- Were the expected outcomes accomplished? If not,
- Was the assessment thorough and complete?
- Did the community or the family participate in formulating the plan?
- Were the problems or issues based on accurate data validated by the community or family members?
- To what extent was the intervention effective?
- Were the criteria for evaluating the plan clear and adequate?
- Was the timing appropriate?

Program evaluation should also include a measure of its relevance, cost efficiency and long term impact (Anderson & McFarlane 1988). This information may be gained from epidemiological data (decreases in morbidity and mortality, or increases in preventive behaviours for populations at risk), or from observation, survey and interview of community residents and other health care professionals working with the community.

Information gained from the evaluation process is then used to reformulate further plans, or to identify successful solutions to problems or issues which may prove helpful in future to the nurse or to others undertaking care of the same individual, family or community. In some cases, this may involve co-ordinating a discharge plan aimed at securing a smooth transition from hospital or health facility.

Discharge planning

Discharge planning is described by Blomquist et al (1988) as 'part of a continuum of care in which those responsible for a client's treatment collaborate in a multidisciplinary team approach to assist the client and family to move from one phase of care to the next' (p. 753). This definition includes movement between all care phases: institution to community; institution to extended or further care facility; agency to agency or community health nurse to family.

The objective of discharge planning is to provide comprehensive (primary, secondary and tertiary) and continuing care. This is achieved by matching community services to client need so that institutional care is shortened or rendered unnecessary. The obvious benefit to the client of non-institutional care, is a more satisfying recovery made in the home or some other more comfortable environment. An additional benefit to both client and the health care system lies in keeping institutional costs down.

Planning for discharge begins with the information gathered upon entry to a hospital or health care resource. This is approached as a collaborative effort between the client and care co-ordinator (usually the primary nurse in the hospital or agency) to encourage client self-responsibility; to ensure a more appropriate health education strategy; and to help the client use the health care system appropriately. The community health nurse *must* be included in discharge planning if it is to be of benefit to the client. In most cases, the onus is on the community health nurse to inform the hospital or health agency of her or his involvement with the client and the extent to which the client is presently utilizing community support services. Providing this information facilitates the co-ordination of client care and helps to prevent duplication of services.

The discharge plan includes subjective and objective information on the problem or health issue; the predicted length of stay in hospital or other facility; the type of environment which the client will be returning to or going to; and the resources which will facilitate ease of transition once he or she is discharged. Information on these resources is usually provided by the community health nurse and includes identifying family and/or friends who will be of assistance, local services, finances, travel, transportation, dietary, and nutritional resources. The plan must also include an estimate of both the current and projected level of care required by the client, and the proposed time frame for moving to the next level of care, whether it be home health care, an after-care program, outpatient follow-up, nursing home care, or attendance at a day care centre (Blomquist et al 1988).

In preparation for release from hospital or the health care facility, a discharge summary is prepared. This contains information regarding the client's basic needs, follow-up appointments, dietary needs, medications, treatments, activities of daily living, and any changes or improvements expected. At this stage, it is important to identify any community agencies involved with the client and family, in order to co-ordinate care and avoid duplication of services. The discharge planning nurse should also gauge the client's attitude towards the discharge, including her or his readiness to assume responsibility for self-care; or his or her attitude towards the person(s) responsible for providing care.

As client advocate, the nurse must be a competent organizer, skilful in communicating with institutional staff, clients, families and other health professionals; and be prepared to liaise with community resources. Although discharge planning is very time consuming, it provides the nurse with the opportunity to enable people to remain in or return to a more health-giving environment; in the larger scheme of things it helps to ensure that the health care system is responsive to community needs.

SUMMARY

The preceding discussion has described the process of nursing the community and managing both oneself and the client population. It is important to note that the nursing process provides a framework for systematizing care rather than a prescription for practice. As a framework it is limited in its oversimplification of nursing a community. For this reason, the steps of the process (assessment, diagnosis, planning, implementation and evaluation) have been elaborated with respect to the author's research findings of how expert community health nurses actually practice in a variety of settings. Examples were also provided to illustrate how the process can be used to guide nursing interventions with communities and families. That aspect of the process which involves identifying and selecting appropriate resources was also described, and the importance of discharge planning was emphasized. The section to follow takes a somewhat broader view of community health nursing in addressing the context of practice.

Study exercises

1. Discuss the criticism that the nursing process is inadequate as a framework for working with families and communities.
2. Describe an example of a community group which would not conform to Maslow's hierarchical model of needs identification.
3. As the nurse responsible for each of the communities/groups listed below, devise nursing care plans for primary, secondary and tertiary prevention for:
   a. A group of women victims of domestic violence in a women's refuge.
   b. A group of adolescents participating in a drug rehabilitation program.
   c. A day care group for the elderly.
   d. A parenting group in a low socioeconomic neighbourhood
   e. A group of male shift workers in a heavy metal industry.
   f. A family comprised of a single mother who works outside the home, two normal school aged children, and a 13-year-old female child with Down syndrome.
4. Construct a discharge plan for an Aboriginal boy of 10 who has been in your care (primarily for home visits to monitor his progress with a severely injured leg) and is now going to the city for reconstruction of his tibia and fibula.

REFERENCES

Alfaro R 1986 Application of the nursing process: a step by step guide. J B Lippincott, Philadelphia

Anderson E, McFarlane J (eds) 1988 Community as client: application of the nursing process. J B Lippincott, Philadelphia

Blomquist K, Stanhope M, Bailey E, Sheahan S 1988 The community health nurse client advocate. In: Stanhope M, Lancaster J (eds) Community health nursing: process and practice for promoting health, 2nd edn. C V Mosby, St Louis, pp 741-759

Burgess W 1983 Community health nursing: philosophy, process, practice. Appleton-Century-Crofts, Norwalk

Clark M 1984 Community nursing: health care for today and tomorrow. Reston Publishing, Reston

Clemen S, Gerber-Eigsti D, McGuire S 1987 Comprehensive family and community health nursing, 2nd edn. McGraw-Hill, New York

Fromer M 1979 Community health care and the nursing process. C V Mosby, St Louis

Higgs Z, Gustafson D 1985 Community as a client: assessment and diagnosis, 2nd edn. F A Davis, Philadelphia

Kenney J 1991 Relevance of theoretical approaches in nursing practice. In: Christenson P, Kenney J (eds). Nursing process: application of conceptual models, 3rd edn. C V Mosby, St Louis, pp 3-19

Lawler J 1991 In search of an Australian identity. In: Gray G, Pratt R (eds) Towards a discipline of nursing. Churchill Livingstone, Melbourne, pp 211-217

Lewin K 1958 Group decision and social change. In: Maccoby E (ed) Readings in social psychology, 3rd edn. Holt Rinehart & Winston, New York

McMurray A 1992 Expertise in community health nursing. Journal of Community Health Nursing 9(2):65-75

Maslow A 1943 A theory of human motivation. Psychological Review 50:370-396

Tripp-Reimer T, Brink P, Saunders J 1984. Cultural assessment: content and process. Nursing Outlook, 32(3):78-82

Turla P, Hawkins K 1983 Time management made easy. Dutton, New York

Yura H, Walsh M 1967 The nursing process: assessing, planning, implementing, evaluation. Appleton-Century-Crofts, New York

PART 3

The context of practice

INTRODUCTION

Communities are enriched or impoverished by the circumstances of the society in which they exist. Political, economic, social and cultural factors combine to provide a unique milieu for the development and maintenance of community health and thus for the practice of community health nursing. Political factors determine the extent to which health care services are made accessible, and define the nurse's role in service provision. Economic factors, in turn, guide political policies which direct resource allocation. Social and cultural factors in a community reflect the myriad of family beliefs, values, attitudes and traditions which both affect and are affected by events, trends and the organizational patterns within and external to the community.

The two chapters to follow provide a starting point for discussion of these contextual factors as they impact on community health nursing. Chapter 5 focuses on the way in which political and economic factors govern the delivery of health care services. Chapter 6 provides some reflections on the family and its effect on both the social fabric and the health of society.

Content: Part 3

5. The political and economic context

A community's health status is profoundly affected by the organization of its health services. The organization of health services is, in turn, dictated by the political and economic processes which facilitate or constrain access to health. If health care is not readily accessible, people are advantaged by neither government benevolence, sophisticated tools and techniques, nor competent and sensitive care givers. One of the difficulties associated with accessing health care is often the consumer's lack of understanding of where, how and from whom services are available. The community health nurse who is familiar with the health care system, and its enabling and constraining elements, can help to provide a better 'fit' between client needs and available services.

HEALTH CARE SYSTEMS

Historically, systems of health care have evolved from local ad hoc measures to contain health problems related to communicable diseases, to organized systems of providing for the complex health and illness needs of rapidly expanding populations. In the UK, the National Health Service (NHS) was instituted following World War II with the objective of providing universal access to health care. It was built on the premise that if health care was accessible, the population's health would improve, there would be a reduction in the need for health care services, and health care costs would ultimately decline (Glaser 1984). The British NHS has undergone several organizational changes over the past fifty years, but it remains a system of government sponsorship in that the government represents the insurer as well as provider of health care. Although the system is centrally planned, budgeting for hospitals and community health services is devolved to the Regional Health Authorities, while District Health Authorities co-ordinate management teams with responsibility for the delivery of local health care. Individuals and families attend a family practitioner who is employed by the local district to provide services to all within a geographically defined area. Once a person is hospitalized, he or she is cared for by specialists employed by the hospital.

Community health nursing in the UK is provided by health visitors and district nurses, some of whom are employed by the NHS to cover a specific geographic area, while others are attached to a general practitioner's practice

(Robertson 1988). Health visitors receive specialized education in community health and undertake an expanded role which encompasses family and community health promotion and illness prevention (Twinn 1991).

Sweden also provides access to health care for all its citizens through an almost completely government operated national health service program. As in Japan, the Swedish system is subsidized by employee health insurance programs (Little 1992). In contrast, the USA has no national health or insurance scheme except for those who qualify for two special government programs: Medicare for the elderly and those with disabilities, and Medicaid for the poor (Little 1992). Although the federal government retains control over public policy and health spending, insurance arrangements for the American system rely on the private sector. Each state has the legal authority to enact and enforce laws which promote and protect health and thus represents the level of management most crucial to the delivery of health care (Hawkins & Higgins 1982). Health care at the local level is primarily dependent on a person's ability to pay either personally or by virtue of an insurance arrangement held by her or his employer. Individuals also have the option of joining a Health Maintenance Organization (HMO) which contracts with the subscriber to provide health promotion and illness prevention programs, and to deliver comprehensive benefits, such as ambulatory and hospital care. However, such organizations also rely on a person's ability to pay a membership fee. Physicians in the USA practise on a fee-for-service basis in the hospital and community alike with treatment costs being met primarily by private insurers (Little 1992).

Community health nursing in the USA is conducted by many levels of nurses in a variety of settings and agencies. These include community health nurse practitioners in independent practice who are reimbursed on a fee-for-service basis; physician assistants who may practise under contract to a clinic or health agency; and community health nurses employed independently or for government (public health) or non-government agencies such as visiting nurse (home health) associations.

The health care systems of Canada and Australia share several common features. Both countries have a system of universal health care insurance (called Medicare in both instances) which co-exists with a parallel system of private insurance. Like the states in the USA and the regions in the UK, provincial health care systems in Canada and state health care systems in Australia represent the critical level of management and delivery of health services. The state (provincial) and territory governments are responsible for public health systems, mental health services, community health services, public health regulations, facility licensing and professional registration (Sax 1989). The federal government in both countries provides grants to the states (provinces) to provide universal insurance coverage, which necessitates ongoing, co-operative federal-state (provincial) planning and consultation. Most recently in Australia, these arrangements have been legitimized by the Commonwealth-State Medicare Agreement covering 1988-93 (Duckett 1992).

In addition to publicly funded care, there has been a recent movement in both Canada and Australia to establish HMOs modelled after those in the USA. Two Australian health insurance companies (HBF and Medibank) have instituted HMOs to provide health promotion and preventive health care to employee and employer groups. However, Biscoe (1989) reports that opinion in Australia is divided as to the the benefits of HMOs. Although their focus (on illness prevention) is admirable, they select out those at highest risk, such as the elderly, thereby defeating the goal of equity in health care.

As in North America, most medical care in Australia is provided by private practitioners on a fee-for-service basis. Although physicians' fees are reimbursed by Medicare, this is not the case with nurse practitioners practising in Australia. As a result, very few nurses practise independently, the exception being a relatively small cadre of midwives. Nurses who practise in Australian communities are primarily employed by state health departments, as community field nurses, school nurses, child health nurses, or remote area nurses. Some are attached to the Royal Flying Doctor Service (RFDS), who, in addition to accompanying clients being evacuated by air to medical facilities, conduct clinics in remote communities with the physicians attached to the RFDS. In an attempt to rationalize nursing services, there has been a trend throughout Australia to appoint generalist community health nurses to a range of positions, rather than perpetuate the demarcations of child health, school health and visiting (field) nurses. As a result, the current role of Australian community health nurses more closely resembles that of their Canadian colleagues who practise as part of the public health system. Others providing community health nursing are those employed by the visiting nurses associations, such as the Silver Chain Nursing Association (in Western Australia) and the Victorian Royal District Nursing Service. Like their counterparts in Canada, (the Victorian Order of Nurses (VON)), Australian home nursing associations have extended the range of services provided, and now focus on health promotion and illness prevention as well as treatment and rehabilitation in the home.

Uniqueness and commonalities

Each nation's health care system is bound to the global health care network by common history and goals. Historically, most first world health care systems evolved from political movements for social reform. Structures, policies and strategies were aimed at overcoming the inequities of health care to the very young, the aged, the poor, the malnourished, the isolated and the diseased. During the post World War II decades, health care programs flourished in keeping with the ideology of social justice and an economic expansionist era. By the 1970s, however, developments in health care world wide were governed by the politics of restraint and cost containment. In the 1990s, health care costs have accelerated to inordinate levels within a climate of global economic recession. Rising unemployment, continuing inflation and a slump in world trade have made restraint and cost containment critical issues. In all countries there is an acknowledged need to develop alternatives to existing cost ineffective health care delivery systems.

Measures intended to increase efficiency and contain costs have resulted in steadily increasing public control over health care. They have also led to attempts to rationalize services, resulting in decentralization of program planning and service delivery. At first glance, the localization of health care looks like a progressive step in making health care more democratic and directed towards the unique needs of the community, however Considine (1992, p. 35) cautions that some initiatives have actually been detrimental to community determined health care. He suggests that regionalization and flattening of the hierarchical structures for health care delivery have reinforced the

> integration and commitment of the corporate management framework through the establishment of an organisationally independent corps of 'generic' or instrumental managers. This group is encouraged to act as a rationalising force, and a battery of evaluation, measurement and reward systems is being developed to encourage and steer them in their work. Local managers can be given far greater autonomy precisely because they can be trusted to support system goals over local priorities and interests.
>
> (Considine 1992, pp. 35-36)

This, and other trends and developments in the organization of health care, have important implications for nursing.

Implications for nursing

Each country's health care system has been designed to meet the needs of the population within the context of the nation's unique, social, political and economic environment, and from the point of view of its ideological orientation. Countries which have provided universal access to health care tend to be underscored by a social welfare orientation, while others are dominated by a competitive ethos. This in turn, is reflected in the organization of nursing services. When nursing practice is predominantly state controlled, there is little room for organizational innovativeness. In the case of a more privatized, competitive system, there is a greater incentive for nurses to adopt a more entrepreneurial approach to practice. Regardless of their differences, all countries have been forced to share common economic concerns, and to review health care policies at all levels. As mentioned above, health care is becoming increasingly guided by a corporatist ethos at the expense of professional input. So how does this affect nursing?

As Baumgart (1988) suggests, individual nurses and organized nursing interest groups should 'examine health care options with a critical and informed eye and participate in the ongoing public debates that surround health issues' (p. 35). In many cases, presenting health care options to clients and families involves ethical considerations, particularly in the case of competing needs and scarce resources (see Ch. 9). If nurses are to contribute to the equitable evolution of health care systems, they must be aware that the world in which nursing is practised is an increasingly political one. Agency politics govern collaboration and delivery of nursing care; local politics influence the organization and accessibility of care; regional politics govern the authorization and jurisdiction of nursing within institutions and community agencies, as well as standards of care giving; and national politics govern the affordability of health care, the legitimate scope of nursing practice and education. Familiarity with the political landscape is therefore essential to the practice of nursing. Nurses must develop political assertiveness and become visible within the system, providing a professional perspective to the 'generic' managers, nurturing informed choice and decision making within their communities. They must gain an understanding of the forces which mould and bind the health care system together, seeking to become informed in order to advocate for the uninformed.

POLITICAL AND ECONOMIC ISSUES IN HEALTH CARE

Politics is defined by Kalisch and Kalisch (1982, p. 31) as the 'authoritative allocation of scarce resources'. Political decisions related to health care are therefore subordinate to economic considerations. According to Aiken (1981) the three major economic issues which impact on health care in the modern world are escalating health expenditures, inflation and the cost-ineffectiveness of health care. Each of these issues warrants careful investigation.

Health expenditures

It is estimated that health care absorbs anywhere from 6% (UK) to 11% (USA) of a country's Gross National Product (GNP) (Little 1992). Holzemer (1992) predicts that this will escalate exponentially to the extent that by the year 2000, the USA will be spending 15% of its GNP on health care. In a market economy one could examine spending in relation to supply and demand, however, the rules of a market economy do not apply to health care for several reasons. Competition lies at the heart of a market economy, and there are insufficient competitors in the health care arena. The medical profession restricts the supply of medical practitioners by controlling licensing, medical privileges and medical education (Sax 1984). The result is a self-perpetuating loop of medical monopoly over health care. This is magnified by the system of reimbursement for medical services by insurance companies. Physicians are reimbursed for services and have no incentive to delegate to non-medical care givers, such as nurses. A further problem lies in the medical practitioners' perceptions of the benefits of medical treatment, which may not be fully informed on the basis of reliable evidence. This often leads to doctors over-emphasizing the relative success of an intervention and the benefits of treatment (Duckett 1992).

Another issue involved in health expenditures relates to the use (or overuse) of services by the public. The issue of whether to curtail seemingly 'free' services for all has been widely debated throughout Australia in the wake of limited hospital beds and a shortage of some specialist services. Duckett (1992) suggests that there are two main strategies being proposed to reduce the role of the public sector in relation to that of the private sector. These include subsidies for private insurance (making insurance contributions tax deductible or rebatable) and limiting eligibility for Medicare benefits. He contends that both these strategies are methods of cost shifting rather than cost containment, the effect being to *increase* rather than reduce health expenditure. He further suggests that such moves will not effect an increase in health services, but would be absorbed in increased administrative costs (Duckett 1992).

It is becoming increasingly obvious that some type of market reform is necessary to slow the escalation of health care costs. Sax (1984) has suggested that if clients and insurers shared the cost of treatment, people may be encouraged to seek out conservative providers. However, economists have attempted to develop a system of evaluating particular interventions by creating standardized measures of disability adjusted or quality adjusted life years (QALYs). To date, these have not proven as useful as expected in that the costs of many interventions have been underestimated (Duckett 1992).

Another counter-argument to medical monopolization is for greater government control over the costs and fees for health care (Sax 1984). However, any argument for greater government control is also fraught with ethical difficulties. Central control of a human service which has to have its greatest skills and commitment at the periphery, risks jeopardizing patient safety in its quest for cost effectiveness (Mustard 1976). The other side of this argument has been rendered more acute by the simultaneous development of high technology medicine and the economic rationalization forced upon most countries by the recent recession. Biscoe (1989) suggests that in this socioeconomic climate we must ask questions such as should all people who may benefit from a heart transplant receive one? Should all AIDS sufferers receive AZT? Should CT scanning be available for diagnosis confirmation in an unlimited manner? Should neonatal intensive care facilities be freely available to all premature babies no matter what their gestation and prognosis? These and other questions relating to resource allocation become vitally important when an inordinate amount of money is being spent on 'high tech' developments while 'low tech' care seems to be devalued in the financial arena. For example, numerous elderly people wait for months for nursing home beds and there are only limited funds available for such things as adolescent suicide prevention programs and research into currently low profile diseases such as multiple sclerosis and asthma.

Leeder (1991) suggests that Australia shares with many other countries the two-edged consequences of medical success in that public demand for health care has now reached insatiable proportions. He proposes that doctors, as a matter of professional duty, must examine the cost-benefit of their practice and participate in broad-based debate about the purpose of the health care system. According to Fyke and Poole (1991), such debate revolves around one of the most pressing ethical issues of the 1990s: the morality of providing an inappropriate or ineffective service when there are unmet needs in society. The most relevant implication for nurses lies in promoting health and/or counselling people towards a variety of health practices. For example, if nurses everywhere urged members of their community to have a cholesterol test and everyone complied, it would cost millions of dollars in lab fees alone. Clearly, issues concerning resources and resource allocation are difficult to resolve in such a way as to satisfy both economists and care providers. Both groups need to work together, sharing their information and heightening awareness in the general public of the implications of health care spending.

Inflation

There are many reasons for the uncontrollable escalation of costs in the health care system. One important factor is the trend toward over-servicing by physicians. This situation is amplified by universal insurance which breaks down financial barriers to care. This is further aggravated by the profusion of costly technological innovations and the fact that the new technologies occur at a time of global population ageing. The elderly incur greater health care expenses than other groups, as they consult physicians and consume more medicines over longer periods of time than younger people. Many are also poor (Sax 1984).

A further inflationary effect derives from the growing trend toward malpractice suits, and the large settlements awarded for successful cases. As a result, physicians tend to practise defensively in a climate of mistrust, often performing more diagnostic tests than are perhaps required. When no rewards are forthcoming for practising conservatively, styles of medical practice tend to be elaborated to absorb every dollar society is willing to spend. Indeed, the Canadian Public Health Association cautions that one of the major threats to universal health care in that country is the $400 million a year of taxpayers' money which is spent on doctors' bills for treatment of the common cold (Mickleburgh 1992). This underlines what many health care professionals already know: most people at any age do not require any form of organized intervention. They need proper housing, income security and informal support from relatives and friends (Illich 1975).

Cost effectiveness of health care

It is widely accepted by care providers that primary health care is the most effective way of securing the health of populations. However, it is financial arrangements, rather than ideology, which propel the system. Cost effective primary health care programs have yet to be demonstrated, and the ability of illness to generate profit remains a major force in determining funding priorities (Olson 1985). Furthermore, there is no consensus on who should provide primary health care, and who should pay for it. To those controlling the funds earmarked for health care, primary health care, which cannot be connected with short term beneficial outcomes, looks like a high-cost alternative.

One impediment to progress in setting up medical networks for primary health care is the maldistribution of physicians. Specialists cluster in urban areas, sustained by insured fee-for-service arrangements. To encourage primary health care practice, the system of reimbursement would have to change to allow parity for wellness as well as illness care. A further impediment lies in the hesitancy of physicians to delegate health care responsibilities to nurses, and the failure of insurance companies to consider nursing services eligible for reimbursement, even those which are clearly more cost effective than physician services. This has resulted in a nursing role which is becoming increasingly disenfranchised, an unseemly irony at such a time when nurses are gaining higher levels of education.

A viable solution would involve establishing the cost effectiveness of well managed integrated community services, wherein the interlinks between community and institutions are maintained, and members of the health care team provide services according to their respective education and abilities. This type of organization would include early discharge programs linked to home care programs, an increase in ambulatory care facilities for the chronically ill and, as Soderstrom (1983) suggests, fewer institutions and curtailment of inefficient technologies.

To date, no one group or political party has a guaranteed formula for efficient and effective health care. However, discussions are being held around Australia on the relative merits of establishing Area Health Boards which would integrate institutional and community services. The policies governing the machinations of these boards have yet to be accepted by all parties concerned, but collaborative structures are being set in place to involve the ideas of consumers, health care providers and members of other sectors, such as environmental and educational authorities.

POLICY FORMULATION

Health is not an international constant. It is shaped primarily by the social, cultural and political environment and personal patterns of behaviour (Milio 1981). Although individuals are free to choose their behaviours, Milio suggests that options are determined by corporate and government policy choices regarding the use of energy, technology, pollution, employment, income maintenance, taxation, pricing, food and agriculture, transportation, housing and health care (Milio 1981, 1985). Achieving health thus depends on a synergy of personal choices by the public, and policy mandates which provide interlinks between all sectors of society (Milio 1981, 1985, Wintemute 1992).

The most politically salient needs which should be addressed by health care policies are those which are associated with client vulnerability: food production, poverty, issues specifically concerning migrants, women and the family, environmental pollution, housing, education, and the equitability and accessibility of health care. Each of these issues are integral to the social fabric of a community. Brown (1992) contends that improvements in the overall health of a community have always come from changes in the social environment. She suggests that co-ordinated social change is needed to advance health and can be achieved through linking education, transport, finance and housing sectors to develop social policies which would provide for such things as subsidized child care and facilities (housing, environmental resources) aimed at enhancing quality of life (Brown 1992). Social policies of this nature represent an attempt at countering the fragmentation which so often occurs in health care systems with an holistic and culturally appropriate approach to health care. To achieve this, policy makers must take into account changing perspectives on societal problems (for example, environmental issues) as well as demographic changes such as population ageing (Howe 1992). Health policies must also correspond to what people want. This may be a long life, or a long life free of preventable disability. Each demands different policy strategies, a different policy 'mix' and different emphasis. The former option has implications for policies which would address primary prevention strategies while the latter shifts the focus to secondary and tertiary prevention (Milio 1985).

THE NURSE'S ROLE IN POLICY DEVELOPMENT

Nurses have an important contribution to make towards health policy planning and development. This can best be accomplished through deliberate and unified strategies. Firstly, awareness of the need for political involvement must be heightened and communicated within the profession. Secondly, a collective base of organizational power must be built. Thirdly, nurses must practise according to a sociopolitical-professional consciousness. Finally, attempts must be made to influence the educational processes by which nurses are prepared for practice.

AWARENESS WITHIN THE PROFESSION:
A RESEARCH PERSPECTIVE

One of the barriers to political consciousness raising in nursing has been the lack of factual, scientifically derived information on issues and trends relevant to nursing and health care policy. According to Gardner and Barraclough (1992, p. 22) 'health policy which is informed by research and which has included the major players in its development, has a greater likelihood of successful implementation'. There is today, a groundswell of nurses asking questions which are politically relevant to community health and community health nursing (Nolan et al 1988, Peoples-Sheps et al 1989, Lipetzky 1990, McGrath 1990, Sharp 1990). The questions are clear, necessary and relevant to the equitable and efficient provision of health care. Although an increasing number of nurses are refining their research skills, exploring new methodologies, and formulating important questions for investigation, many researchable questions remain, including the following:

- Which clients typically seek care from nurses? from physicians? from other care givers?
- Which clients utilize community outreach programs?
- What are the health outcomes of these choices?
- What variables affect adoption of suggestions for health maintenance?
- How do cultural issues impact on health status?
- What factors influence a client's ability to become actively involved in choosing health care alternatives?
- Which changes in consumer behaviour are related to social and economic trends? to availability of services? to personal and cultural variables? to health care insurance? to changing population needs? to national health care goals?
- To what extent is disempowerment a precipitating factor in illness?
- How cost effective is community health nursing care? under what circumstances?
- How well do community health nursing courses prepare for the realities of practice?

The initial most important question to ask is: How can these research questions be addressed and who will help? Communication difficulties associated with isolated practice settings seem to have interfered with progress in building a body of community health nursing research. Isolating attitudes have also contributed to this situation. Many rank-and-file nurses view research as an elitist conspiracy; the concern of nurses who have moved out of the practice setting. Research reports are often couched in jargon unfamiliar to all but the scientist, leaving the importance of their findings either misunderstood or ignored. In addition, many of the questions pertinent in a community health setting require an interdisciplinary approach. Information relevant to community health practice may come from such other health disciplines as public health administration, occupational health and safety, health economics, political science, social work, behavioural science, and women's studies. Often the person who can act as a resource in accessing such information is in an educational setting, and would welcome dialogue with those in practice.

To encourage research among practising nurses, networks for collaborating and sharing must be established, possibly through departmental or professional interest groups. Within a network, nurses and other health care professionals with research skills could offer suggestions to systematically explore research questions, and provide assistance in interpreting the results in a clear and meaningful way so that they could be communicated to others. This type of mentoring would offer an incentive to practising nurses who are often the first to speculate on the impact of trends or developments in health care, but have not had the opportunity to develop the skills to systematically explore issues as they arise.

One of the most important steps in the entire research process is the dissemination of findings. A wealth of research information remains tucked away within specialist areas, hidden in academia, or otherwise detoured on its way to the practice areas. Steps to overcome this include having someone within a local nursing network 'flag' and/or condense current journal articles or new research findings for distribution to other members. This works well within interest groups affiliated with state, provincial or district nursing organizations. Usually such organizations have at least one member who has ongoing access to this information. Local health departments often provide a similar service. In areas where no such service exists, the onus is on individual nurses to make contact with colleagues in universities and/or local hospitals and health agencies.

Increasing specialization in nursing has led to professional fragmentation by function at a time when nurses need consolidation of efforts. Aroskar (1980) cautions that such fragmentation contributes to nursing's 'fractured image'; an image which erodes the credibility and effectiveness of the profession. One way of countering this situation is for nurses to commit themselves to professional unity and professional empowerment.

BUILDING A POWER BASE

The word 'power' is used in a multitude of ways in our society, but, quite simply, can be defined as the ability to affect something or be affected by something (Kalisch & Kalisch 1982). Empowerment is the enabling of power, or control, and self-empowerment is securing or enabling of self-control. Kalisch and Kalisch (1982) identify two subcategories of power as authority (the right to expect or command obedience) and influence (persuasion and/or manipulation).

Power, authority and influence, the tools of the political process, are fundamental to the practice of nursing. Authority structures are a given in nursing, even with the flattening of hierarchies which has accompanied the decentralization of services. Influence is also second nature to nursing, as witnessed by the persuasive tactics commonly employed to encourage healthy behaviours. Both authority and influence can be used in the political forum to empower the nursing profession. To do this, nursing must recommit, redefine and repolish its professional identity, adopting a role which links professional, political and social advocacy as convergent strategies toward community self-empowerment (see Fig. 5.1).

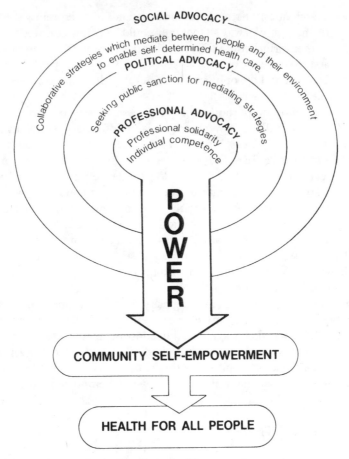

Fig. 5.1   The diffusion of power in primary health care nursing.

PROFESSIONAL PARTICIPATION

Activities which contribute to the nursing power base include participation in professional organizations, networking and mentoring. Involvement in professional organizations is the most important link to the profession, and to presenting a unified and politically interested image to the public. As well as disseminating research information, nursing organizations represent a vehicle for collecting and distributing political information, such as legislative news on issues relating to health care, and the voting behaviours of elected representatives. Some professional organizations delegate members to liaise with government agencies and elected officials for this purpose. Other information distributed through nursing organizations includes the names, position description, purpose and location of nurses in senior government positions, the identity of nurse legislators and elected representatives, and the names of government officials sympathetic to causes concerning nurses and health care.

In many parts of the world, nurses have formed political action committees, often as a subgroup of their local professional organization. The objectives of such groups range from gathering and distributing information on political issues which impact on nursing, to encouraging nurses to take a more active role in politics, to lobbying for passage of desired legislation and defeat of undesired measures, to supporting candidates for public office. Some political action committees have specialist subcommittees, such as those which provide expert testimony for committees and commissions that are considering health related legislation (Ellis & Hartley 1988).

Networking

Nurses can also make a political impact by participating in public campaigns for social action, most of which are aimed at advocating for groups who have been marginalized within their own social and political system. Social actions are typically based on principles of equity, self-determination and self-help, and thus are compatible with nursing goals for primary health care. Australian examples include the campaign to promote social benefits and social acceptance for separated mothers and their children, the movement for the ordination of women priests in the Anglican Church, the campaign to get child abuse on the political agenda and the lobby for the Royal Commission into black deaths in custody (Baldry & Vinson 1991). By getting involved in social issues, nurses are able to share their professional power with others. Networks can be cultivated with conservation groups, anti-nuclear groups, women's issues and self-help groups, lobby groups for anti-pollution and anti-smoking bylaws, and groups concerned with such issues as neighbourhood safety or landlord-tenant arrangements. When nurses individually and/or collectively establish contact with such groups the profession becomes better informed and strategies to improve health become appropriate, current and unified.

One additional way in which nurses can have an impact on the political agenda is through formal special interest groups concerned with advocacy for vulnerable people. For example, the Public Health Association of Australia, a non-political organization which represents more than 40 public health disciplines, has instituted 11 special interest groups (SIGs) whose members (including nurses) have contributed to as many policy statements on issues ranging from Aboriginal health to tobacco advertising.

Mentoring

Peer supervision and collaboration on projects or planning committees strengthens subgroups of nurses, creating units for collective action. When a unified voice is needed on an issue, it is important to know the extent of collegial strengths and peer support. A considerable amount of influence is also exerted through the mentoring process. Malone (1984) explains that the mentor's role is to provide a safe space for the mentee's career to grow, through direct access to information, by providing advocacy on issues, and by extending reflected power. As Puetz (1983) suggests, the mentor links the novice to the realities of practice, therefore, the role modelled by one politically conscious generation of mentors has the capacity to empower a second such generation.

Individual action

For those who are unable to participate in group activities for political action, alternative measures can be taken toward individual and professional empowerment. These include reading nursing and health related newspaper and magazine articles with a political focus, and keeping up with current issues identified in the nursing literature. Dialogue with other politically conscious health professionals also enhances political sophistication, and helps to consolidate efforts toward building a power base.

There are ways in which individual community health nurses can both lend and receive visible and meaningful social support. Many issues arise in the press begging for a letter to the editor. These may relate to school health programs, cuts in day care spending, landlord-tenant policies or discrimination issues. Although it is commendable to respond as a socially conscious individual, a letter signed by a 'concerned member of the nursing profession' is a nobler gesture, as it advances the image of nursing as a politically aware profession. It is unfortunate that when nurses as a group are mentioned in the press, it is usually (and judgementally) in respect to industrial action instead of social action. Similarly, letters to one's member of parliament (MP), member of the legislative assembly (MLA), Congressman or Congresswoman gather import when they are declared as authored by a professional nurse.

Nurses have traditionally conformed and over co-operated with others, and have failed to be assertive enough to capitalize on the power they hold (Burke 1979). Some of the reason for this can be attributed to the way in which we have been socialized. Baumgart (1980) suggests that as (primarily) women, nurses have not been socialized into the political role, and therefore require such 'repair' programs as assertiveness training. Organizational circumstances have also prohibited empowerment to some degree, but in the community, this is gradually changing with the extension and expansion of the role as co-ordinator of care and advocate for community change.

Despite our socialization and organizational constraints, Labelle (1986) delineates ten levers of power which nurses have close at hand. These are:

- Nurses provide care at all levels
- They work in all settings
- They represent the largest category of health workers
- In most countries, nurses have organizational structures

- They are in direct contact with the population for extended periods of time
- Nurses possess and control massive amounts of information
- They are frequently the main connection between the individual, the family and other health professionals and agencies
- Nurses have competence, knowledge and specialized skills
- They have access to communication channels
- Nurses vote.

To nurture community self-empowerment, nurses must serve as role models, making their expertise visible, graciously accepting and utilizing their professional power through socially and politically conscious practice strategies.

POLITICAL AWARENESS AND NURSING PRACTICE

How is nursing practised according to a social and political consciousness? What are the modes, or styles of practice, and what are the individual behaviours which typify sociopolitical professional practice?

Nursing practice is defined by the requirements of the profession; the demands of a particular position; the context in which practice is conducted; system and/or economic constraints; the limitations of time; expectations of the employing organization and individuals to whom the nurse is responsible; and the personal and professional characteristics of the nurse. Political action is modified by any or all of these factors. However, in any practice situation, there are ways in which political awareness serves to enhance practice strategies.

The following illustrations are presented as an attempt to debunk the assumption that 'playing politics' is either too complex, or that it is beyond the scope of normal nursing practice.

Case 5.1: An occupational health issue

An occupational health nurse was hired by a private, unionized corporation to provide a health service for 'all company employees'. The position description included maintenance of general health and safety; treatment of occupational and non-occupational illness and injury; periodic health assessments; and several target programs, such as hearing conservation, employee fitness, and employee assistance programs for substance abuse. The company had many female employees whose escalating absenteeism rates corresponded to a community-wide decrease in availability of day care services. The women individually, and through their union, approached the nurse about getting involved in their struggle to have the company provide day care facilities. As a politically informed professional, the nurse understood the relationship between the mothers' economic situation and their health. Clearly, the nurse knew she must advocate for an improvement in working conditions regarding day care, but not to the extent of jeopardizing the women's employment status, or diluting her own image as advocate for all employees. The context of an industrial setting demanded a practice style which would not distance the nurse from either labour or management groups. The company management was not previously aware that the occupational health nursing role included any involvement with the social and economic welfare of the workers. This had to be diplomatically suggested to them at a time when they would be receptive to the idea. The manager responsible for the occupational health centre held a narrow, traditional view of the nursing role, and furthermore, had no sympathy for 'women who take up men's jobs!' The nurse therefore had to both gain and give respect, by acknowledging his point of view, but also had to be resourceful enough to prevent his attitude from obstructing further channels of authority which might be of help in resolving the problem. It was becoming obvious to the nurse that the company needed a policy to deal with the day care issue. One feature of this company was that employees benefitted from annual profits through a profit sharing scheme, but only when economic targets were met. The nurse therefore needed to gain access to the financial status reports and economic forecast, so that a realistic appraisal could be made before a policy was planned. This particular occupational health nurse had previous experience in the field, well developed communication skills, and a working knowledge of production industries. From the time she was hired, she determined to become familiar with the company's organizational structure, priorities and dynamics; to identify the influential individuals within both management and labour groups; and to project an image of herself as competent, caring, trustworthy and authoritative. The nurse's strategy in this situation included the following steps. She documented the concerns of the workers regarding the lack of day care facilities, and their inability to find child care alternatives. She then requested a report from the municipality on the distribution of day care centres in the area. She wrote a letter to her local member of parliament to inquire about the existence of a working group addressing the day care issue. She contacted her local community health nurse colleague to ask whether she too,had been involved in activities aimed at securing day care facilities and suggested an alliance of efforts. Together they composed a thoughtfully worded letter to the editor of the local paper mentioning the changing needs of a community which now contained more separated parent and working mother families than previously, and querying whether the community should be demonstrating a commitment to helping these people. The occupational health nurse then drafted a note to the occupational health nurses' interest group to include the issue on the agenda for their next meeting. Her next step was to graph absenteeism rates among female employees with pre-school aged children for the time period since local day care facilities had closed. Once this was done, she requested an appointment with the company's manager of human resources to discuss the issue. Upon receipt of the evidence identifying a need for day care provisions within the company, the human resources manager struck a working committee to write a policy proposal to be presented to the union and management groups. The nurse volunteered to join this committee, and during one of her lunchtime information sessions with the employees, relayed the information that she and others in the company were engaged in a committee to review the entire issue. The employees were heartened, and the situation was temporarily defused. Over time, and with much revision and negotiation, the policy was ratified by the company.

Political struggles do not succeed or fail based on the logic of their case (Fatin 1987). There was logic on both sides of this case: to maintain the health of the workers on the one side, and production schedules on the other. The outcome of this particular struggle may not have been as positive had the nurse not been able to cultivate co-operative relationships within the company and build a base of support from her colleagues.

Politics in health care, and therefore in nursing practice, consists of exercising power, consolidating power, and affecting a change in power relationships (Baumgart 1980). In this case, the nurse affected change by perseverance and consolidating power. She gained power by empowering others, accepting the orthodoxies and protocols of the workers, the company, her peers, the media and the politicians. It is a prescription for practice with no guarantees. But when it works, no matter how long it takes, the rewards are immeasurable.

Case 5.2: Agency politics and the remote area nurse

A state health department nurse was engaged in delivering primary health care to a remote desert community of nomadic indigenous people. During the three years she was in this community, she came to know the culture and the people. Most of her clients lived in the area surrounding her town site for approximately four months of the year, then moved on in a relatively predictable fashion to several other 'home' camps. During the times when the people made their home in this community, they brought their children to the nurse for examinations and immunizations; occasionally came by for advice; and often, to have transient illnesses treated. In the distant city, the press had recently created a furore out of the revelation that nuclear deposits from weapons testing during World War II had been found in one of the neighbouring camp sites. The nurse had read the newspaper reports with interest, and received reassurance from her district supervisor that she would be notified if there was to be any increased health screening and surveillance, or special treatment protocols for anyone suffering ill effects of radiation exposure. The supervisor also promised to send her all the relevant literature on health risks associated with nuclear wastes. In the meantime, state health authorities were looking to the federal Aboriginal medical services agency for direction. News of the discovery had filtered to all the desert people through their informal networks, and the elders of the group approached the nurse, asking for comment on the rumour that they may be forced to relocate forever. The nurse promised to gather all the information she could and report back to them. Telephone calls to the community services and education departments, both of whom were involved with the group, proved fruitless. Neither department had received confirmation or denial of the relocation, or had been given guidance from the federal Aboriginal authority. Without warning, two social science researchers arrived at the nurse's home, the only permanent residence in the town. They produced a written authority to conduct a study of the impact of recent events on the group's migration patterns. The nurse offered them lodging, only to learn that they were only the first of several 'expert' teams arriving in town to conduct environmental and social impact studies. During the ensuing week, the city people arrived, camping within the nurse's compound, and began their studies.

This coincided with a boycott of the nursing station by the Aboriginal people. No one requested treatment; no scheduled child health visits were kept. When the nurse arrived at the school to help prepare the soup for the children's lunch, she was told that they had eaten, and her help was not needed. It was obvious to her that the trust which had previously bonded her to the group, had been violated. Her requests to the city people to leave the village were greeted with accusations of anti-intellectualism and largely ignored. A telephone call to her supervisor elicited sympathy, but no action to have the outsiders removed, as they had all been granted permission to be there by a higher authority. The nurse's solution was to write a letter to the following: her supervisor; the social scientists and teams of experts; the department of community services; the federal Aboriginal authority; the federal government departments conducting the impact studies, and to her state nurses' association. In the letters, she identified herself and briefly described her position, and the lines of authority within her department. She provided a brief overview of her role with the Aboriginal people followed by a statement of concern that, based on specified changes occurring among the people, intrusion by the white community may have jeopardized the ongoing health of the people. Her letter requested that information on the issue, its seriousness and any planned intervention, be sent to both her and the elders of the group. Finally, she identified all the others to whom she had written, so that each would see the seriousness, and acknowledge the legitimacy and appropriate channelling of her efforts. The issue became a 'political football', bouncing between state and federal government departments, various concerned official agencies, consumer groups, and the press. By the time responses were received by the nurse, the Aboriginal group had moved on. Over the next few months, a quarantine was placed on the area suspected of harbouring the hazardous waste, and the Aboriginal camp site was relocated. Guidelines for medical surveillance were issued by the federal health agency, but no clients presented for examination. All attempts by the nurse to contact members of the group failed, as they had elusively 'gone bush'.

This scenario illustrates the profound effect that cultural and agency politics have on the provision of primary health care. There are times when it is not enough to be familiar with cultural issues; when it is necessary to encourage or even coerce others into doing so as well. These activities fall within the scope of social advocacy, and therefore must be considered as an integral part of the co-ordination of client care.

Population-focused community health nursing is intensely political, whether it be practised in remote or populated regions. Political networking provides the nurse with a lifeline to those with the power to either enable, or constrain practice. At times, it can mean the difference between health and illness for the client population; and at times, be a deciding factor in whether the nurse is able to cope or gradually becomes professionally disengaged. In the above example, the remote area nurse displayed the courage of her convictions and persevered with the political process until the situation was defused and the time was right to begin to rebuild her relationship with the Aboriginal people. These types of nursing actions do not come about by accident. To prepare for community health nursing, with its political ramifications, nursing education must play a critical role.

THE ROLE OF EDUCATION

If nursing is to be practised in a sociopolitical professional context, a strong commitment is required from nursing educators in both academic and practice settings. The university provides an ideal climate for the political education of nurses, as universities often provide the backdrop for social change (Fagin & Maraldo 1981). However, efforts toward resocializing the profession must involve collaboration between practitioners and educators of both preservice and continuing education programs. Education for the future must broaden students' perspectives of world health concerns and strengthen their commitment to resolving global health problems (Fagin & Maraldo 1981). Health care politics, economics, technology, leadership and management skills must be simultaneously incorporated into the curricula and modelled within the health care system.

Political awareness can be fostered in students by having them observe the legislature in action, particularly when health care issues are discussed; participating in official and non-official organizations involved in improving health care; attending nursing organization meetings; and becoming actively involved in the delivery of health care services within the educational institution (Torres 1975).

Through visible involvement in current issues, conducting in-service sessions, and continuing to practice, educators have the opportunity to enlighten students at the same time as contributing to the reunification of educators and service providers (Kramer 1985, Kernen 1985). Obscuring the boundaries between the two groups presents several desirable political outcomes. Education and service can conjointly develop health policy that considers professional nursing services a major component of the promotion and maintenance of health in the population. When both groups collaborate in policy making within the work setting, they can publicize and articulate the value of professional nursing services, rather than allowing their goals and skills to be devalued and stereotyped (O'Rourke 1981). In this way, the classroom is taken into the community practice setting, and paves the way for complementary political and professional roles to become normalized. Furthermore, the interpersonal skills of both groups are strengthened by participation in organizational strategies, conflict resolution and the management of health care (WHO 1984, Haggerty Davis & Posey Deitrick 1987).

SUMMARY

Health care has become increasingly political. For the nurse to function as a co-ordinator/partner in community health care, it is necessary to understand the system within which health care is delivered, particularly the political machinations which impact on her or his ability to advocate for the community. It is of concern that nurses, the largest group of health care workers in the world, are often excluded from health care decision making and policy development. For nurses to become politically involved necessitates heightening awareness of political issues within the profession, building a base of organizational power, practising according to a sociopolitical consciousness, and attempting to influence the educational processes which prepare nurses for practice. For some nurses, political action groups provide access to political involvement, while for others who may be unable to participate in collective action, individual efforts form their contribution. All nurses can, to some extent, become politically active through practice strategies which are underscored by political awareness. In addition, all nurses can contribute to building bridges of tolerance within and between the profession. Education, though not a panacea, is a perfect place to begin. Practice that is interesting, relatively autonomous yet connected and helpful in attaining health for all will be its reward.

Study exercises

---

1. Identify three important things you would need to know about the health care system if you were to relocate from a community health nursing position in Australia to one in another country.
2. Describe the steps you would take to increase your community health nursing colleagues' awareness of one of the following political issues:
   a. a proposed development in your city of an industry which will potentially emit high levels of toxic waste
   b. discriminatory practices in your local community.
3. Once you have encouraged heightened awareness among your professional colleagues on either of the above issues, what further steps could be taken to effect a positive outcome?
4. Identify the major areas for policy development in your community.
5. List five obstacles which nurses must overcome to participate in developing social and/or health policies.

REFERENCES

Aiken L 1981 Health policy and nursing practice. McGraw-Hill, New York

Aroskar M 1980 The fractured image: the public stereotype of nursing and the nurse. In: Slicker S, Godow S (eds) Nursing image and ideals: opening dialogue with the humanities. Springer, New York

Baldry E, Vinson T 1991 Actions speak. Longman Cheshire, Melbourne

Baumgart A 1980 Nurses and political action: the legacy of sexism. Nursing Papers, Winter:6-16

Baumgart A 1988 Evolution of the Canadian health care system. In: Baumgart A, Larsen J (eds) Canadian nursing faces the future. C V Mosby, Toronto, pp 19-37

Biscoe G 1989 The future: planning, reformation, uncertainty. In: Gray G, Pratt R (eds) Issues in Australian nursing 2, Churchill Livingstone, Melbourne, pp 83-97

Brown V 1992 Health care policies, health policies or policies for health? In: Gardner H (ed) Health policy: development, implementation and evaluation in Australia. Churchill Livingstone, Melbourne, pp 91-117

Burke S 1979 Why nursing has failed. In: The emergence of nursing as a political force. National League for Nursing Pub. no 41-1760, New York, pp 57-64

Considine M 1992 Policy: managed or expert? In: Gardner H (ed) Health policy: development, implementation and evaluation in Australia. Churchill Livingstone, Melbourne, pp 29-50

Duckett S 1992 Financing of health care. In: Gardner H (ed) Health policy development, implementation and evaluation in Australia. Churchill Livingstone, Melbourne pp 137-161

Ellis J, Hartley C 1988 Nursing in today's world. Lippincott, Philadelphia

Fagin C, Maraldo P 1981 Health policy in the nursing curriculum: why it's needed. National League for Nursing Pub. no 15-1845, New York

Fatin W 1987 Nursing and the politics of health care. Paper presented at the thirty-fourth oration and investiture of fellows and members of the New South Wales College of Nursing, Sydney

Fyke K, Poole B 1991 Doing the right things. Policy Options, Oct. 11-12

Gardner H, Barraclough S 1992 The policy process. In: Gardner H (ed) Health policy: development, implementation and evaluation in Australia. Churchill Livingstone, Melbourne, pp 1-28

Glaser W 1984 Health politics: lessons from abroad. In: Litman T, Robins L (eds) Health politics and policy. Wiley, New York, pp 305-339

Haggerty Davis J, Posey Deitrick E 1987 Unifying the strategies of primary health care and nursing education. International Nursing Review 34(4):102-106

Hawkins J, Higgins L 1982 Nursing and the American health care system. Firesias Press, New York

Holzemer W 1992 Linking primary health care and self-care through case management. International Nursing Review 39(3):83-89

Howe A 1992 Participation in policy making: the case of aged care. In: Gardner H (ed) Health policy: development, implementation and evaluation in Australia. Churchill Livingstone, Melbourne, pp 237-271

Illich I 1975 Medical nemesis: the expropriation of health. Pantheon, New York

Kalisch B, Kalisch P 1982 Politics of nursing. Lippincott, Philadelphia

Kernen H 1985 The merging of education and practice. In: Stewart M (ed) Community health nursing in Canada. Gage, Toronto, pp 592-601

Kramer M 1985 Why does reality shock continue? In: Comi-McCloskey J, Kennedy-Grace H (eds) Current issues in nursing, 2nd edn. Blackwell, Boston, pp 891-903

Labelle H 1986 Nurses as a social force. Journal of Advanced Nursing 11:247-253

Leeder S 1991 Ailing system needs more than economic treatment. The Weekend Australian, Sept 7-8 Melbourne, p 19

Lipetzky P 1990 Cost analysis and the clinical nurse specialist. Nursing Management 21(8):25-28

Little C 1992 Comparison of national health care systems. Nursing & Health Care 13(4):202-203

McGrath S 1990 The cost effectiveness of nurse practitioners. Nurse Practitioner 15(7):40-42

Malone B 1984 Strategies and approaches to policy making: a nursing perspective. Occupational Health Nursing Jan:24-27

Mickleburgh R 1992 Medicare dollars poorly spent, group contends. The Globe and Mail, Sept, 17, 8

Milio N 1981 Promoting health through public policy. F A Davis, Philadelphia

Milio N 1985 Creating a healthful future. Community Health Studies IX(3):270-274

Mustard J 1976 Towards an understanding of the health delivery concept. In: Murray J (ed) Health care delivery systems in North America: the changing concepts. University of Windsor, Windsor, Ontario, pp 1-6

Nolan J, Beaman M, Sullivan J 1988 Activities and consultation patterns of nurse practitioners with Master's and certificate preparation. Public Health Nursing 5(2):91-103

Olson K 1985 Economic resources and restraints. In: Stewart M (ed) Community health nursing in Canada. Gage, Toronto, pp 114-128

O'Rourke M 1981 Health policy: the clinical perspective. National League for Nursing Pub. no. 15-1846, New York

Peoples-Sheps M, Efird C, Arden Miller M 1989 Home visiting and prenatal care: a survey of practical wisdom. Public Health Nursing 6(2):74-79

Puetz B 1983 Networking for nurses. Aspen, Rockville

Robertson C 1988 Health visiting in practice. Churchill Livingstone, Edinburgh

Sax S 1984 A strife of interests. George Allen & Unwin, Sydney

Sax S 1989 Organisation and delivery of health care. In: Gardner H (ed) Politics of health: the Australian experience. Churchill Livingstone, Melbourne, pp 225-250

Sharp N 1990 What will physician payment reform mean for nurses? Nursing Management 21(10):16-17

Soderstrom L 1983 Taxing the sick: health policy at a crossroad. Canadian Centre for Policy Alternatives Pub no. 11, Ottawa

Torres G 1975 Offering learning experiences that reflect the changing role of the professional nurse. In: The changing role of the professional nurse: implications for nursing education. National League for Nursing Pub. no 15-1574, New York, pp 27-33

Twinn S 1991 Conflicting paradigms of health visiting: a continuing debate for professional practice. Journal of Advanced Nursing 16:966-973

WHO 1984 Education and training of nurse teachers and managers with special regard to primary health care. WHO Technical Report Series 708, Geneva

Wintemute G 1992 From research to public policy: the prevention of motor vehicle injuries, childhood drownings, and firearm violence. American Journal of Health Promotion 6(6):451-464

6. The family

INTRODUCTION

The social context of a community is a reflection of the relationships shared between people and their environment. The uniqueness of the family in this context lies in its role as gatekeeper between individuals and the society in which they live. That is, the family acts as a filter interpreting and mediating attitudes, beliefs and values back and forth between its members and the wider social community. As the basic unit of society, the family represents the cornerstone of community health. Within the family can be found both causes of and solutions to health problems, and a rich spectrum of behaviours and strategies which contribute to the evolution of society. It is vital, therefore, that nurses practising in the community are familiar with the social issues and trends which impact on the family as well as the ways in which changes in the family affect society.

DEFINING THE FAMILY

The family can be considered as a social system comprised of persons who co-exist within the context of expectations of 'reciprocal affection, mutual responsibility and temporal duration' (Wright & Leahey 1987, p. 7). Such a definition makes allowance for families 'to define "family" for themselves, and to act on valued relationships even when they do not arise from blood ties, marriage, legal adoption, or common residence' (Wright & Leahey 1987, p. 7). This concept of family reflects enormous changes in societal attitudes, values and norms from when the family was considered an intact nuclear unit of mother, father and children all living together and adopting traditional roles where father was the breadwinner, mother looked after the home and children and the children were seen but not heard.

THE FAMILY IN SOCIETY

The family as an entity has changed considerably from the days when it was primarily considered an economic unit, and it is important for those involved in promoting health within families to understand how society has influenced the changes and how the family defines itself and interacts with others. For example, economic resources, determined by society, is the most important issue affecting families today. Poverty is linked to a range of family problems such as inadequate parenting and family homelessness which have become pervasive social problems (Moccia & Mason 1986, Halpern 1992, Berne et al 1992). By exploring the societal forces, traditions and roles which create the meaning of health and illness, the individual and family may be able to work towards securing opportunities for improved health and may be freed of the isolation and alienation that accompanies individual problem ownership (Butterfield 1992).

Up until the age of industrialization, the 'family farm' was the backbone of society, and family relationships revolved around maintaining the solidarity which would make the family economically viable. Since that time, the family has steadily diversified in response to major social, economic and political changes. These changes can be linked to historical events. The wars precipitated entry of women into the work force. Away from the protected home environment, many women began to demand greater rights in society; the right to vote and to participate in shaping the social forces within which their children would be reared. The dawning of the information age and improved communication brought about a global awareness of alternative family mores and lifestyles. Marriage is now only one of many options which include living alone, cohabitation, maintaining a sexual relationship while living separately, living with peers, or delaying marriage until later life or until pregnancy (Edgar 1991). In some cases, these choices have enhanced the quality of life of family members, while in others, the result has been family dissatisfaction and disharmony. Today, many families find themselves in the process of questioning and redefining their role in contemporary society and this has very strong implications for all health care professionals attempting to guide them. It is therefore imperative that nurses working with families gain an appreciation of the changes confronting the family in today's society and the issues which society must deal with as a consequence of these changes.

The most dramatic demographic changes in the family have included the escalating rates of divorce, the blending of families through remarriage, a decline in those choosing to marry, marriage being delayed, and smaller numbers of children per family (Eastman 1989). Other changes include longer life expectancy, marriages in which child rearing dominates only a small percentage of the life span, and the three or four generation family. Eastman (1989) suggests that these changes, combined with changes in societal attitudes towards marriage, mean there is little legal or social coercion on couples to remain married. This may be either good or bad, depending upon whether the stable patterns of the past were, in effect, merely masking hidden difficulties. Despite the traumas which change often brings, current patterns may hold the potential for a more free, more fully human concept of marriage and family life (Eastman 1989). In any event, the separated family is a phenomenon of contemporary life which must be acknowledged.

The separated family

With the rapidly rising rates of separation and divorce, the separated family has become increasingly visible in today's society. In the past, there was a certain stigma attached to divorce, and such families were considered the scapegoat for any child behaviour which failed to conform to traditional expectations. Throughout the 1950s, 1960s and 1970s, whenever a child of separation or divorce misbehaved, it was customary to blame her or his behaviour on the fact of having come from a 'broken home'. An accumulating body of social research has now identified the importance of societal influences on the family. As Duffy (1992, p. 330) reports 'the influences of economics, social supports, and sex-role attitudes on the health of women heading one parent [sic] families and their children are enormous'. Current societal attitudes are also shifting towards acknowledging variability rather than conformity in families' behaviours, attitudes, beliefs and values. The 'broken home' is a dysfunctional and discriminatory label which points to neither cause nor effect and fails to capture either the essence or dynamics of separated families. The term 'single parent family' is similarly stigmatizing. To call a family where one parent has moved from the home and who maintains an ongoing relationship with the children a single parent family negates the ability of the visiting parent to assume a warm and nurturing parental role. Research conducted between 1960 and 1980 pointed towards negative outcomes for children of divorce on such variables as achievement at school and social competence (Institute for the Development of Educational Activities and National Association of Elementary School Principals 1980); however, today this is not considered to be the norm. An Australian study comparing general competence of children who came from intact and separated families indicated that living in a one parent household was no barrier to achieving a high level of general competence (Amato 1987). This concurs with the findings of Wallerstein and Kelly (1980) who suggest that the crisis of parental divorce sometimes acts as a spur to children's development and may result in superior competence in some children.

One of the most crucial outcomes of separation and divorce is the financial cost to families and society itself. Eastman (1989) reports that the total annual cost of marriage breakdown and divorce in Australia is in the realm of $1900 million. This works out to $175 per head of population, only 44 cents of which is allocated to family guidance and other support systems aimed at preventing marriage breakdown. Many separations result in poverty, particularly for women and children. Eastman (1989) cites research which indicates that 75-80% of women are significantly worse off after marital separation, and that the average fall in income is around $80 per week. She reports that 'one parent families [sic] are six times as likely to be living below the poverty line as are two-parent families' (p. 104). Furthermore, marital separation often begins a cycle of intergenerational poverty, as McCaughey's (1987) study of family support networks in Victoria suggests.

In addition to financial costs, the emotional and social costs of separation and divorce are significant. Despite the fact that many couples separate because of intolerable stress in the family, the stress following separation and divorce is often overwhelming. A large body of evidence suggests that many separating parents become preoccupied with their personal grieving and go through a period where they provide less than satisfactory support for their grieving children (Hetherington et al 1977, Burns 1981, Furstenberg & Nord 1985). Some children are catapulted into adulthood prematurely, particularly in cases where there is role reversal and the child adopts the supportive role for the grieving parent, at the expense of resolving his or her own grief. Family therapists call this the 'parentified child' (Eastman 1989, p. 108). Wallerstein and Kelly (1980) suggest that the most critical time in a child's adjustment is during the first year following the separation. During this period the child needs to work through the trauma of loss of the parent who has left the home and begin to adjust to such things as new family roles, relocation and/or changed financial status.

One group which has thus far been the subject of very little research following separation and divorce is the non-custodial parent. Despite the need for children to have the influence of both parents, many non-custodial parents lose contact with their children over a period of time (Burns 1981, Furstenberg & Nord 1985, Weitzman 1986). Weitzman (1986) suggests that as nurturance of children receives no protection in the law, and as women continue to have custody but insufficient financial resources to care for them, non-custodial parents may choose to become less invested in children. This trend is already occurring in Australia. The author conducted a study in 1991 of non-custodial mothers in Western Australia which revealed that a lack of financial resources is indeed the most significant factor influencing the mothers' ability to maintain a warm and nurturing relationship with their children, and often the precipitating factor in the mothers' decision to relinquish custody (McMurray 1992b).

Nursing implications

Marital separation and its aftermath is a highly emotional time of turbulent change for most people and, although some families are able to move beyond the crisis stage fairly quickly, others remain traumatized for extended periods of time. For the community health nurse, the range of psychological and social issues affecting the family's health and potential for growth present a unique challenge. In many cases, the nurse becomes involved with the custodial parent and her or his child(ren) through child health visits or in the school health clinic. The presenting issue may be a child's behaviour problem, or a school child's inability to cope with studies. Often the child is seeking a replacement for the attention which has ceased since the absent parent left the home. Alternatively, young children may develop illnesses precipitated by the stress of the separation. In some cases, the parent is having difficulty coping with the home situation, and comes to the nurse seeking help for himself or herself. The nurse's initial task is to assess the situation with respect to whether a referral is necessary. The family may need social welfare programs or ongoing counselling and the referral can be dealt with in an uncomplicated manner. In some cases, the parent may be seeking ongoing counselling from the nurse because of a previously established relationship of trust. According to community health nurses interviewed in one study, this is problematic because of time constraints and the lack of educational preparation for family counselling (McMurray 1991). However, many nurses are able to provide at least initial counselling, guidance on issues related to child health and development, and appropriate referrals to agencies providing social and psychological services.

The care giving family

Another important family phenomenon relates to the family caring for a member with a disability or chronic illness. With the increasing proportion of elderly people in today's society, many families are called upon to provide extended periods of care for a family member and to assist with decisions related to health and medical care (Glasser et al 1992). The importance of the family in caring for elderly members will become more pronounced over time because of the trend towards encouraging family self-care in the home, for both economic and ideological reasons. Anderson (1990) suggests that the ideology of self-care has placed enormous pressure on families to care for their ill, elderly or disabled members at home. She explains that, although encouraging independence and self-care is admirable and empowering for the sick individual, health care professionals may 'fail to recognize the complex factors that influence people's management of illness in daily life' (p. 72). She urges that nurses and others involved in planning for self-care in the family attempt to understand the extent to which the mediating circumstances of people's lives influence their ability to assume self-responsibility for health. In addition, O'Neill and Sorensen (1991) suggest that it is important for nurses co-ordinating home care to examine the changing type and degree of care giving burden placed on family members related to prognosis. These authors recommend, for example, that research be undertaken into the burden of care experienced when caring for a frail, demented elderly family member as compared to a family member who has the potential to return to some degree of health and resumption of previous family roles (O'Neill & Sorensen 1991).

Nursing implications

Wright and Leahey (1987) cite Strauss and Glaser's list of tasks that families of chronically ill patients must perform, and identify nursing implications for each. The first is crisis prevention and management. Family members must learn to anticipate any crisis which might be expected in the case of, for example, cardiac conditions, severe diabetes and epilepsy. The nurse's role is to provide appropriate information to help the family recognize changes in the individual's condition and to respond appropriately. The second major family task is regimen management. The family must become familiar with the health routine and their role(s) in maintaining that routine, as well as familiarizing themselves with the role of the nurse when intervention is required. A third task is symptom control which requires that the individual and family rely on their own judgement, wisdom and ingenuity. The nurse's role in symptom management is to educate clients about signs, symptoms and their possible outcomes. Fourth, families must adjust to the temporal and role disruption which accompanies chronic disease, and be helped to explore ways of dealing with changing circumstances. This is particularly important in the case of mothers with chronically ill children. Turner-Henson et al's (1992) research revealed that the heavy burdens and constraints facing mothers of chronically ill children have a significant influence on mothers' caring and parenting behaviours, as well as limiting opportunities for family interaction.

A fifth issue relates to families learning to handle the disease course or trajectory, a task which the nurse can help with by providing anticipatory guidance, particularly in the case of terminal illness (Wilson 1992). The sixth major task involves overcoming social isolation, which may be caused by the client's reduced energy, impaired body functioning, disfigurement, time consuming medical regimen, and possible desire to hide the disease and its management. The nurse can help by encouraging family members to seek respite from the caring process. The final task is to secure funding for treatment and daily needs in the face of partial or discontinued income. The nurse's role is one of advocacy, helping family members to explore options and making referrals to the appropriate social services. For all of these major tasks the most effective techniques for helping families adapt to the situation involve organization, family co-operation and evaluation of consequences (Wright & Leahey 1987).

Watson (1992) delineates the many strains which occur in families in response to the burden of caretaking. She suggests that frequently, resentment, compounded by guilt feelings occurs, and contributes to the family's social isolation. Although many families appear to adapt effectively, health care professionals 'seldom recognize the effort put forth to achieve this' (p. 55). The primary task of the health professional is thus to ensure that all assessments are family-centred, and that preconceived notions of the family's needs are set aside until family members have had an opportunity to identify priorities for care and support from *their* perspective. O'Neill and Sorensen (1991) contend that to understand both the carer and care recipient's perspectives, nurses must undertake research studies which will examine family dynamics and recipient responses to family care giving.

For the nurse visiting the family, understanding the ambivalent feelings which individuals may have is the first step in advocating for *all* family members. For example, when a family member is ill over a long period of time, family members may devise a roster of times when each can help with care-giving tasks. In some cases, circumstances change, and the *types* of tasks (cooking, arranging for services) as well as the *timing* of tasks may change. Unless there is ongoing discussion of the care-giving process, individuals may become increasingly stressed and exhausted, to the point of becoming unable to cope (Wilson 1992). One or another family member may continue to fulfil his or her obligations without respite to avoid upsetting the ill person or causing other family members undue pressure. In the extreme, this situation has the potential to cause the entire family to become dysfunctional. The home visiting nurse is often in a position to gauge the situation and to facilitate family problem solving.

In guiding the family towards self-support, the nurse should try to encourage a non-judgemental sharing of feelings and concerns so that family members can explore a range of options and develop a plan for care-giving. This helps each member to explain her or his individual strengths, limitations, and expectations for the future, issues which some families take for granted and thus fail to articulate. The family plan must also be steered towards accommodating to the changing needs of the ill member. This is particularly important at the tertiary (rehabilitation) stage of illnesses which are not of a chronic nature. For example, in a study of adjustment following heart attacks Johnson (1991) described the importance of family dynamics during the rehabilitation process. She reported that when families were able to co-operate, supporting and respecting each other's needs, rehabilitatees felt encouraged and cared for, which enabled them to develop a sense of trust in themselves, and ultimately a sense of self-control.

The multiproblem family

Another major phenomenon in working with families concerns what many community health nurses have come to describe as 'the multiproblem family'. In some respects, the term seems to be an indictment of families whose circumstances have led them into a cycle of help-seeking. For example, the migrant, mother-headed family living close to poverty and caring for a chronically ill family member may be considered as having multiple problems. Often, however, the multiproblem family is one which has a history of being unable to cope with any set of circumstances; that is, it is a disempowered family. Such families present an enormous challenge to community health nurses and other health professionals.

Nursing implications

Lynch and Tiedje (1991) describe the multiproblem family as sharing certain defining qualities. Although they vary in size, composition, location and the nature of problems they present, their problems are both internal and external, they cut across social, economic and health contexts, and they are known for chronicity and crisis. These authors suggest that, in order to deal effectively with such families, nurses should come to terms with three major aspects which affect the way they relate to the family: value conflicts, control issues, and information exchange. They present an argument pertinent to the nurse-client relationship, suggesting that the middle class outlook of many nurses contributes to their ineffectiveness with multiproblem families. This may derive from four main value sources; Judeo-Christian doctrine, which places responsibility on the 'haves' to help the 'have-nots'; democratic idealism, with its moral imperative that God helps those that help themselves; the Puritan ethic which posits that character is everything and circumstances are nothing; and social Darwinism, which dictates that the strong survive and the weak perish. Superimposed on these values are the Nightingale values of cleanliness, conformity, cheerfulness, efficiency and moralizing. Lynch and Tiedje (1991) advise that recognition of these values is the first step towards understanding how to intervene successfully with multiproblem families as an enabler for family empowerment.

Carey (1992) identifies the goal setting process as paramount to intervening with multiproblem families. She suggests two alternative approaches. First, the nurse should ask the family what they want or need to work on. Next he or she should help them break down the problem areas into manageable subproblems in order to prioritize problems, clarify goals and establish feedback points which can provide opportunities for positive reinforcement and serve as signposts as to when to start working towards a new goal. In less functional families which do not have the ability to identify needs and/or to ask for specific kinds of help, the nurse should share her or his assessment and diagnosis with the family, suggest possible goals, then check to see if the family wants to work towards the goals or set different ones. In any case, the role involves acting as an information source, facilitating the goal setting process, providing guidance in locating and using common resources, and advocating for community health services (Carey 1992).

The following case study illustrates how a community health nurse must adopt a client-centred approach in order to provide information, guidance and advocacy for the multiproblem family.

Case 6.1: Working with a multiproblem family

The family was visited because there had been many problems which the nurse first became aware of a few weeks earlier when the woman gave birth to twins. The mother was living with a de facto husband who had recently been severely injured in an industrial accident and had been hospitalized for several months. The relationship was going through a difficult time. There was no day care facility available for her 3-year-old and her 15-year-old daughter was pregnant. The family was also having major financial difficulties since the husband's injury. The nurse explained to the woman that she was visiting to check on the twins' developmental progress. During the visit the nurse attempted to gain a sense of how the family was coping by inquiring about the well being of all family members. She felt that the mother was anxious to discuss some particular issue which wasn't forthcoming during the process of conducting the babies' assessments. Instead of terminating the visit on completion of the assessments she refocused the mother's attention on the 3-year-old and discussed some alternatives for child care. She then attempted to redirect the conversation towards the family's preparation for the birth of the 15-year-old's child, and offered to have a chat with the daughter about antenatal care and her relationship with her boyfriend. Once she had reassured the mother that she would help counsel her daughter, the nurse asked the mother if there was anything she could do to help her secure additional finances, mentioning a supplementary mother's allowance scheme which had been recently initiated. Finally, the nurse suggested the mother just relax for a moment and try to think of any other issues she would like to discuss. Once the mother turned her thoughts from the myriad of problems affecting the children, she was able to discuss her feeling of utter exhaustion and need for temporary respite. She revealed to the nurse that the major problem she had been trying to avoid concerned her obligation to visit her husband in hospital and to decide whether she wanted to preserve the relationship or not. The nurse allowed her to express her feelings, which she had been setting aside in the face of all the other problems, then suggested that once she had the 3-year-old in day care, she leave the twins with the 15-year-old and attend a family counselling session. The nurse guided her through her priorities. She could not attend to her need for marriage counselling (the most worrisome need from the mother's perspective) until she had organized the younger children's care. Together the nurse and the woman explored the options, discussed the need for the mother to clarify her personal, as well as family, goals, and established a plan for the nurse to revisit and monitor progress. Although the nurse's approach was to view the family holistically, she had attempted to guide the woman through each problem separately, to facilitate clarification and prioritization of goal setting, and to collaborate with the woman to establish a plan for follow up visits where she could provide the woman with reinforcement and review her, and the family's progress.

(From McMurray 1991, p. 207)

Although the nurse working with families must understand the practical interface between family health care and illness, it is important to link nursing activities to the theoretical and conceptual bases for practice (Wright & Leahey 1987). A systematic approach can then be adopted to investigating the reciprocal and interdependent relationships which exist between individuals, their families, and the groups, communities and societies to which they belong. The discussion to follow thus describes three commonly used theoretical approaches to the study of the family in order to provide a perspective for the process of family nursing.

THEORETICAL PERSPECTIVES OF THE FAMILY

Systems approach

The systems approach conceptualizes the family holistically as a whole system with interdependent parts. The system and its parts have both structural and functional components. Friedman (1986) explains structure as the arrangement and organization of parts, while function relates to its purposes or goals, and is the outcome of structure.

The family can be viewed as an open system, one in which material, energy and information is exchanged with the environment. Family functioning is therefore affected by what is occurring in society. Similarly, the individual's functioning is affected by what is occurring in the family. Because the family is dynamic and ever changing it, in turn, impacts on society, providing the impetus for societal change and growth.

As a system, the family is characterized by non-summativity, that is, the whole is greater than the sum of its parts. The characteristics and qualities of that whole derive from the interrelatedness of family members; as Minuchin (1984) describes it 'like chips in a kaleidoscope', contributing to the pattern of the whole (p. 3). Similarly, the family can be likened to a child's mobile. When one part is touched there is a rebound effect to all others.

The family is part of a hierarchy of systems, such as the community-family-individual hierarchy, and the grandparent-parent-child hierarchy. Those systems which lie in its immediate environment have more impact on the family than those in the more distant environment. For example, the sibling subsystem affects family functioning to a greater degree than the extended family, or grandparent subsystem.

The family system is also characterized by family boundaries which are more or less permeable, selectively opening and closing according to the family's needs. Boundaries serve to promote adaptation and differentiation of the various family subsystems, such as the spouse, parent-child, sibling and extended family subsystems. A balancing of roles within these subsystems serves to promote family adaptation and homeostasis. In response to input, Friedman (1986) suggests that the family and its members adapt by either accepting or rejecting incoming information, energy or services, or by modifying the input to meet its needs.

Energy exchange is an important characteristic of all systems. When there is a positive energy contribution to the family's adaptation, the family can be thought of as energized. The energized family, according to Pratt (1976), is characterized by the following:

- interaction by all members, regularly and in a variety of contexts
- maintenance of varied and active contacts with a wide range of other organizations and groups to enhance and fulfil the interests of its members
- active attempts to cope and master living by joining groups, seeking out information, discovering options and making decisions
- a fluid internal organization with flexible roles, responsiveness to change, shared power and autonomy and growth of its members.

Such a family energizes its subsystems and suprasystems as it is energized by them. This feedback mechanism produces a circular paradigm of family adaptation within its structural-functional framework as illustrated in Figure 6.1. The systems approach is therefore useful as a guide to analyze the family over time and through changes.

Structural-functional approach

While the emphasis within a systems approach is on the whole, the structural-functional approach focuses more on a linear parts analysis of the family (Friedman 1986). Both orientations address the family as a social system with functional requirements which make it congruent with society. Friedman identifies four basic structural dimensions which are interrelated and interact to organize the family. These include the family's role structure, value systems, communication processes and power structure.

Role structure

Role structure includes positions within the family and their associated roles. For example, wife-homemaker and husband-wage earner are positions and primary roles in the traditional nuclear family structure. Each role is

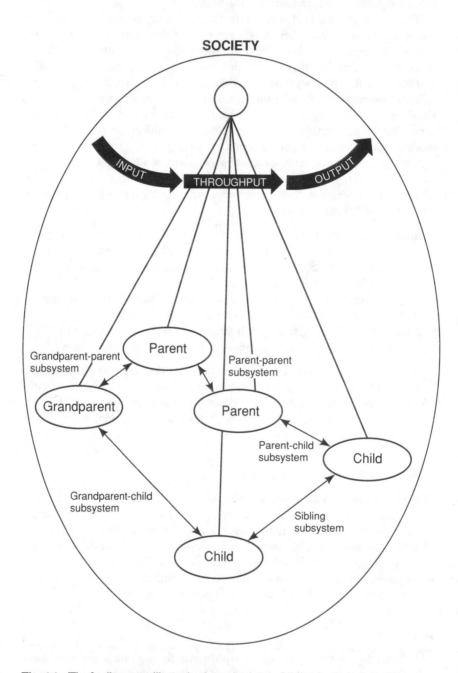

Fig. 6.1 The family system illustrating input (society to family member), throughput (family member to family member via subsystems) and output (family to society).

characterized by relatively homogeneous and predictable behaviours, although to a lesser extent today than in the past. For example, Australian men in the past were 'shackled by a traditional view of fatherhood' which precluded them being involved in the social processes surrounding pregnancy and birth (Pease & Wilson 1991, p. 58). Today, many fathers participate in the birth event to the extent that some families accept this as a normal part of a father's role.

In the majority of families, the wife and husband play several formal roles: marital, parenting, recreational, housekeeping, kinship, therapeutic and sexual roles. When the number of family members is small, opportunities and demands exist for each member to play several roles at different times (Friedman 1986). This is particularly true in separated families where one parent functions as caretaker and children often contribute to the family's economic and domestic tasks.

In addition to formal or overt roles, family members also perform informal roles in order to meet various emotional needs. For example, one family member may play the role of family 'coach' or encourager, while another may play the 'martyr', or 'scapegoat' (Satir 1967).

Family values

The second structural dimension is that of family values. A family's values, comprised of ideas, attitudes and beliefs, guide the development of family norms or rules. The family's values are a composite of societal values and the culturally determined value systems which individuals bring to the family from their family of origin. Edgar (1991) suggests that the construction of family themes or cultures over time 'depends critically upon the relationships between generations via property and wealth transmission, reproduction and socialisation and the passing on of cultural themes and stories' (p. 5). Family values include such things as productivity and achievement, materialism, work ethic, education, equality and tolerance of diversity (Friedman 1986).

Family communication

Family communication processes represent the third structural dimension. Information that is passed between family members enables individuation (developing a sense of self), the development and maintenance of self-esteem, learning about other people, and learning to make choices (Friedman 1986).

Many of the family's affective needs are met by the capacity for creative, open, tolerant communication patterns. Optimal communication occurs when the message is clear, the content and affect (the words and music) are directed from the sender through clear channels, and the receiver understands the message without ambiguity or confusion. Healthy families relate with this level of openness, and do not hesitate to communicate emotions, displaying a full spectrum of feelings both verbally and non-verbally (Wright

& Leahey 1984). According to Friedman (1986), the family which is communicating positively demonstrates mutual respect for each other's feelings, thoughts and concerns, spontaneity, authenticity, and constructive conflict resolution.

Family power structure

The final family structural dimension rests in the power structure of the family. Family power is revealed through the communication patterns of the marital, parental, offspring, sibling and kinship subsystems. Friedman (1986) identifies types of family power ranging from the chaotic or leaderless family to one in which there is marked dominance, or absolute control, by one family member. Egalitarian or functional families are those with flexible structures for sharing power among family members and complementarity between partners. Minuchin (1974) adds that healthy families have a clear and functioning hierarchy in which the parents and children have different levels of authority.

As mentioned previously, the consequence of family structure is function. Duvall (1977) lists six major functions of the family which balance individual and family roles. The most important of these is that of generating affection between family members. A second function is to provide the stability and continuity which fosters emotional security for family members. Third, the family gives satisfaction and a sense of purpose. A fourth function is to provide continuity of companionship. The fifth function is to provide socialization and social status, which is at once ethnic, racial, national, religious, economic, political and educational. A sixth family function involves inculcating controls and a sense of what is right. The family passes along the rules, rights, obligations and responsibilities essential to the survival of society. To Duvall's list, Friedman (1986) adds the reproductive function, to ensure continuity, and the health care function, as it is within the family that most health care needs are provided for.

This list of family functions is neither static nor exhaustive. At times, the family serves to fulfil a broad range of functions to varying degrees. Furthermore, the extent to which one family function is fulfilled is often dependent upon satisfactory fulfilment of other family functions, situational variables, the family's evolving structure, and its developmental stage.

Developmental approach

The developmental approach suggests that families go through stages of relative stability which are qualitatively and quantitatively different from adjacent stages. Developmental theorists study the family's interactions and relationships at the various stages and as they change over time. At each stage of the family life cycle, certain developmental tasks are expected to be achieved to meet the family's biological requirements, cultural imperatives, aspirations and values. Duvall (1977) identifies eight stages and their correspondent tasks as follows:

Stages of family development

Stage 1: Beginning families—the stage of marriage. At this stage the family's three main developmental tasks include establishing a satisfying marriage or relationship, relating harmoniously to the kin network, and family planning.

Stage 2: Early child bearing—the stage of parenthood. Developmental tasks at this stage centre on establishing the young family as a stable unit, reconciling conflicting developmental tasks of family members, and jointly facilitating achievement of individual developmental tasks to strengthen the family as a whole.

Stage 3: Families with preschool children. At this stage, the family is concerned with adjusting space and living arrangements, protecting the children from illness and injury, integrating new members into the family, socializing the children, and learning to separate from the children as they prepare to go to school.

Stage 4: Families with school children. Developmental tasks of this stage include, as at other stages, maintaining a satisfying marital relationship, and promoting the children's school achievement.

Stage 5: Families with teenagers. The task of maintaining a satisfying marital relationship remains a primary developmental task at this stage. In addition, open communication becomes a priority at such time as the values, life styles, moral and ethical standards of both parents and adolescents may be challenged by one another.

Stage 6: Launching centre families. As children leave home, the family attempts to encourage independence and to expand to include new family members by marriage. The shifting roles of parents at this stage provides freedom to rebuild the marital relationship and to assist ageing or ill parents of either spouse.

Stage 7: Families of middle years—postparental stage. Developmental tasks important to this stage include maintaining a sense of physical and psychological well being through a healthy environment, sustaining satisfying relationships with children and ageing parents, and re-strengthening the marital relationship.

Stage 8: Families in retirement and old age. The tasks of this final stage of development include maintaining comfortable living arrangements, adjusting to a reduced income, maintaining the marital relationship or adjusting to the loss of a spouse, and maintaining intergenerational family ties.

The developmental approach provides a useful yardstick for anticipatory guidance through the family's stage-related challenges and issues. Identifying discrete stages does however, neglect to address the overlapping issues of the family in two or more developmental stages at once, and the between stage events which allow a family to change (Friedman 1986). A further limitation lies in assuming a relatively homogeneous and stable family form which is not the usual case in separated families.

Stages for the separated family

For the separated family, Johnson (1988) suggests two developmental stages in addition to Duvall's.

Stage 1: Establishment of the single parent family. Tasks related to this stage include developing new patterns of power, communication and affection, altering child rearing patterns, developing new social networks, fulfilling physical maintenance tasks, and coping with disrupted intimacy and sexual aspects of the marital relationship.

Stage 2: Custodial parent continuing, instituting or reinstituting an occupation. At this stage, tasks include developing new family maintenance arrangements, both physical and affectational, maintaining family morale, nurturing family members and re-establishing or maintaining self-esteem through outside involvement.

Stages in remarriage and the blending of families

Carter and McGoldrick (1980) identify developmental issues related to remarriage and the blending of families, which would add three more stages:

Stage 3: Entering a new relationship. The critical task for this stage would be recommitment to marriage and forming a new family.

Stage 4: Conceptualizing and planning the new marriage and family. Tasks at this stage include working at openness in the new relationships, planning for maintaining co-parental relationships with ex-spouses, planning to help children deal with fears, loyalty conflicts and dual family memberships, and realignment of relationships with extended families of ex-spouses to maintain connections with children.

Stage 5: Remarriage and reconstitution of the family. Following the formation of the new family, relationships within the family must be realigned, boundaries must be restructured, relationships with ex-spouses and extended families maintained and memories and histories shared to enhance step-family integration (Carter & McGoldrick 1980).

All three perspectives of the family (systems, structural-functional and developmental) provide a useful framework for assessing and planning nursing interventions which will help a family to meet its health needs.

THE HOME VISIT

In most cases, family nursing activities occur in the context of a home visit. The nurse's self-management activities are undertaken prior to the actual visit. Following this stage, client management is begun, which involves establishing contact/rapport, screening (in some cases) and interviewing family members as the initial step in family assessment. There are several advantages to conducting a family assessment in the home. One advantage is that information on family structure and behaviour may be more accurate when obtained in the home setting. Observations made in the home environment help to identify both barriers and supports for achieving family health promotion goals. In addition, family members often feel a greater sense of control in their own home, and may be more receptive to the idea of active participation in meeting their health needs when they are interviewed at home (Carter & McGoldrick 1980). Five phases of a home visit are outlined by Loveland-Cherry (1992):

1. Initiation of a home visit

Before a family is visited, the nurse seeks to clarify the source of the referral and the purpose of the visit.

2. The pre-visit phase

Whenever possible, the nurse should make a courtesy telephone call to the family prior to the visit to establish rapport, introducing herself or himself, identifying the reason for the contact, explaining how the family came to be referred, and scheduling the visit. A brief conversation with family members helps to clarify issues and needs and serves to encourage their input into planning. During the conversation, the visit can be planned for a mutually convenient time and duration, and when as many family members as possible are available. The telephone call can be terminated with a review of the time, place and purpose of the visit, and provision of a contact number where he or she can be reached. If the family has no telephone, a postcard or letter may be used to notify the family of the intended visit. Following the pre-visit contact, family records or discharge plans and referral documents should be reviewed in preparation for the visit (Carter & McGoldrick 1980).

3. In-home phase

During the interview, the home visiting nurse should be sensitive to potential negative concerns of the family related to the visit. Some families are reluctant to warm to a violation of their privacy by a representative of a public agency 'checking up on them', or to having their home and lifestyle judged by a member of another class and/or culture. Consequently, much of the initial visit may be taken up with establishing the relationship and conveying a sense of genuineness and respect for the family. Once the nurse has introduced herself or himself to the family, a brief social conversation may help to defuse anxiety and prepare for a more indepth assessment interview.

Wright and Leahey (1984) suggest that the family interview be a circular process, with family members being encouraged to discuss their perceptions of what is occurring in the family rather than simply answering direct, linear questions. By encouraging family members to discuss their concerns in their own words, the nurse becomes aware of cues which form the basis for judging family needs. Judgements can then be validated by asking the family members to confirm his or her judgements, and to collaborate in setting priorities for care. During the interview the nurse may also become aware of the family's metaphor; its characteristic way of conceptualizing events and issues (Wright & Leahey 1984). At this stage, the nurse actively listens without taking notes, so as not to erect any paper and pencil barriers to communication. Following the family's discourse, the nurse may suggest that together they summarize what has been discussed, and explore any other existing issues which may require attention. At this point, an assessment guide can be produced and shared with the family.

A useful guide to assessment must provide for assessing the family system with its structural-functional arrangements and its developmental stage and tasks. Friedman's family health assessment form represents an example of such a tool (see Appendix 3).

Family identification data is collected first, followed by the developmental stage and history of the family. At this point, it is helpful to draw a genogram of the family to provide a visual representation of the family constellation (see Fig. 6.2, 6.3). Most families are intrigued by this process and if it is convenient, enjoy receiving a copy of their completed genogram. Following this, data are collected on family functions and family stressors and coping mechanisms. Finally, the nurse and family member or members collaborate on generating a list of family strengths and areas for improvement, as a basis for planning.

Throughout the assessment process, the influence of family culture must be assessed. Although family roles, values and beliefs may shift and change with time, and as members move in and out of the family, they are primarily ascribed by culture, and are manifest in caretaking, communication patterns, and in political, economic, religious and health care practices (Carneiro 1985). As Butrin (1992) proposes, nurses need to understand the cultural context which contributes to each family's uniqueness. For this reason, Leininger's (1978) nine major cultural domains can be used as an appropriate framework to be incorporated into the assessment process. They include:

Cultural life patterns or lifestyles. This includes living arrangements, food and eating habits, clothes, celebrations, sleep, the expression of affection, the significant others, and ways of greeting or addressing others.

Values, norms and expressions. Within this domain are religious and family planning practices, and norms for acceptable behaviour of family members and others coming into the home.

Cultural taboos and myths. These include behaviours related to illness, death, disasters and any behaviours which are forbidden.

World view and ethnocentric tendencies. This category includes opinions on the world in which the family lives, events occurring in that world, and attitudes toward outsiders.

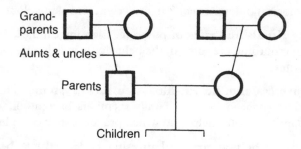

Fig. 6.2 Blank genogram (From Wright & Leahey 1984).

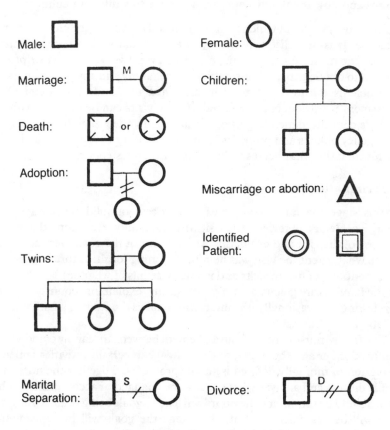

Fig. 6.3 Symbols used in genograms (From Wright & Leahey 1984).

Cultural diversities, similarities or variation. Included in this domain are such biological differences as height, weight and skin colour.

Life-caring rituals and rites of passage. Lighting candles, giving gifts, grieving and mourning are some of the behaviours which reflect a culture's rituals and rites.

Folk and professional health-illness cultural systems. This involves the behaviours engaged in when family members become ill, such as to whom the family goes for help, and which practices they consider helpful.

Specific caring behaviours and nursing care, values, beliefs and practices. Childbirth practices, feeding, nurturing and caretaking are included in this category.

Cultural change and acculturation aspects. Included in this domain are those strategies which are used to adapt to a change in job, school, roles, groups and how the family copes with a move to a different country.

A family assessment which includes cultural aspects represents a very rich database. It is unrealistic, however, to expect that such a comprehensive assessment must be carried out in one or even two visits. It is helpful to attempt to obtain general information on the family and any pertinent issues or problems during the first visit, and then to decide how detailed an assessment is subsequently required. Future visits can be planned with the family's consent, depending upon family needs, their eligibility for service and agency politics and priorities (Loveland-Cherry 1992). Once a plan for the future visit(s) has been set the termination phase begins.

4. Termination phase

At this stage the nurse completes the process of validating and setting priorities. He or she reviews the visit with the family, reiterating the goal or purpose of the visit and evaluating whether or not the goals were achieved, and to what extent the visit was helpful. Planning for the future begins with the scheduling of future visits and includes details of what needs to be done for the family (care giving, advising, reassuring, explaining, counselling and/ or referring). Occasionally, the intervention takes the form of a family-nurse collaborative contract.

The family-nurse contract is an agreement between the family or individual family member and the nurse, to each engage in certain activities aimed at resolution of mutually defined issues or problems. Together the nurse and family discuss and analyze what needs to be changed or accomplished, what goals should be set, what behaviours will lead to goals being fulfilled, how the plan will be evaluated, and at what stage the goals will be renegotiated (Loveland-Cherry 1992). Through contracting the nurse relinquishes the therapeutic relationship, allowing the family control over its health care decisions. One area where a family contract has proven most helpful is in helping families facilitate weight control in an adolescent member. Many school health nurses see young girls, in particular, who need help with weight control. The nurse's approach is typically to collaborate with the girl to plan a contract which includes enlisting the help of the physical education teacher to set a program for physical activity; negotiating with the parents for positive reinforcement of small changes (compliments, encouragement) and restriction of availability of high calorie foods; and drawing up a schedule for weight checks and discussion of progress. The contracting strategy can be either very successful or totally inappropriate, as in the case of a family which is unable or unwilling to take responsibility for health care decisions. Once a contract is established and/or a plan for the future outlined, the termination phase is considered completed.

5. Post-visit phase

Responsibility for the home visit does not end until the interaction has been recorded and referral documents completed. Documentation procedures will usually be determined by the agency to which the nurse is attached. To these records may be added the family genogram, any written contracts and recommended strategies for subsequent visits, referrals or follow up surveillance.

The nurse may also want to include a family ecomap (Fig. 6.4) in the record. As with a genogram, the ecomap provides a visual summary of

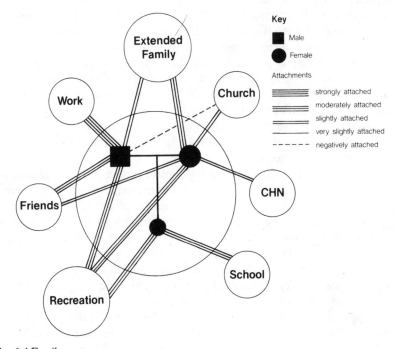

Fig. 6.4 Family ecomap.

information gained during the assessment, the genogram providing historical information, and the ecomap depicting family members' contact, attachments and conflicts with their suprasystems (Wright & Leahey 1984).

NURSING THE FAMILY: A RESEARCH BASIS FOR PRACTICE

As the previous discussion indicates, families provide an interesting challenge for community health nurses, in both their multidimensional nature and the uniqueness of their health problems and concerns. In a study of expert community health nurses conducted by the author, nurses practising in school health, home visiting and child health were asked to comment on the role of the family in their practice activities. All participants declared that, irrespective of job description or subspecialty area, they considered themselves to be practising family nursing (McMurray 1992a). Some of the findings of that study are presented here to paint a picture of community health nursing practice at the expert level and to illustrate the extent to which nursing the community is nursing the family.

BACKGROUND TO THE STUDY

Benner's (1984) seminal work on clinical expertise suggested that many accepted models of nursing practice are limited in their capacity to explain how nurses *actually* practice when they get to the stage of being experts in their field. According to Benner and others researching the area of expertise, experienced nurses often achieve a comprehensive assessment without consciously applying a 'process'. These nurses seem to have a finely tuned ability to pick up on cues in the client encounter situation by critically reflecting on their intuitions. Intuitive thinking is the product of deep situational involvement in a nurse-client encounter to the extent that one develops a 'gestalt' about the situation (Benner & Tanner 1987, Dreyfus & Dreyfus 1986, Pyles & Stern 1983, Rew 1988). Over time there is an accrual of knowledge which becomes incorporated or embedded into the nurse's skill repertoire, particularly in making clinical judgements. Situations are judged for their individual circumstances, but in relation to prior experiences through a process Schon (1983) calls 'reflection in action'. Twinn (1991) suggests that this ability to use intuition in making clinical judgements illustrates professional artistry in nursing. Others have called it clinical expertise (Benner 1984, Benner & Tanner 1987).

Benner's (1984) research suggested that clinical knowledge develops from a complementary synthesis of both perceptual and analytic knowledge and, although analytic knowledge can be taught in a classroom, perceptual knowledge must be acquired by practice or the next best thing, which is to observe or listen to experts describe what and how they actually perform in practice situations. Benner's rationale for her research provided the stimulus for devising a study to examine the processes of community health nursing practice (McMurray 1991). This study was based on the premise that the most accurate and germane information about community health nursing would come from those judged by their colleagues to be expert practitioners. The investigation was thus based on reputational sampling, where a group of senior community health nurse clinicians and supervisors were asked to nominate expert practitioners from within their respective districts. Those nurses identified as experts subsequently agreed to be observed in practice situations and interviewed on their particular strategies and reflections on community health nursing practice.

THE EXPERT COMMUNITY HEALTH NURSE

The expert community health nurse seems to move confidently between the stages of self-management and client management and demonstrates a finely tuned ability to pick up on cues in the client encounter situation. As with Benner's (1984) experts, community health nurses who participated in the study described a deep understanding of client situations in terms of intuitive hunches. A school health nurse explained this process in the context of an encounter with a young girl who she had recently been concerned about: 'I knew there was something going on there...something in her body language told me something else was going on...a little bit of eye evasiveness, pale face, something about her that wasn't quite right' (McMurray 1991, p. 197).

This nurse acknowledged the importance of acting on her intuitive hunches which became more frequent the longer she had been in practice. Many other nurses explained that although they assess situations systematically, with experience, they had learned to trust their intuitive judgements. The two vignettes to follow provide examples.

Case 6.2: Intuitive judgement: a home visiting episode

I'm knocking on the front door of a house that I've never been to before and there's no answer. I go around to the back door and bang loudly to no avail. I know an elderly man lives there, but there is no sign of anyone. I notice there's a pile of clean clothes with a note attached near the back door so I know someone's called in recently. I decide to visit the neighbours who seem to know my client, and no, they haven't seen him. 'Something' tells me that I should persevere and keep knocking and calling out and try to see inside which is impossible due to the cluttered state of the house. The place is completely locked up. After another 10 minutes of calling out and knocking I finally get an answer. The elderly man I've come to see says he's O.K., just having a rest. After questioning him further he tells me he's on the floor, doesn't know how long he's been there and doesn't want to move but he'll be O.K. and 'come back later'. Thinking he's had a fall and injured himself and been on the floor all night I tell him I have to get in to see him and seeing as everything's locked I'll have to get the police to come. 'O.K.' he says, reluctantly. I call the police from the neighbour's phone and they come and get into the house by cutting the fly wire off a window and we find my client on the kitchen floor, unable to move with a painful right hip. He's in unkempt clothes and has been incontinent. I ask the police to call an ambulance and he goes to hospital and is diagnosed with a fractured neck of femur. Why keep knocking, persevering, checking all avenues? Because 'something' tells you something's wrong.

(McMurray 1991, pp. 209-210)

Case 6.3: Intuitive judgement in a school health episode

I was involved in a child abuse case. It was difficult because DCS (Department of Community Services) was changing social workers and trying to get one who wasn't afraid to go into the home. It was so frustrating. I knew a 5-year-old was being sexually abused and that her brother was being beaten but there wasn't enough proof, and this man had been in every state and DCS had a huge file on him. He kept threatening to go to the press so the social worker needed to be very gutsy and very sure of her judgement. Finally, we persevered and succeeded in having the children removed from the home. Originally, I knew intuitively that there was something wrong with the kids. There are classic symptoms, pale, furtive glancing, being withdrawn etc., but it was more than that. It's like a look in the child's eyes and you just know by looking at them that something is going on with them. You learn to see that with experience.

(McMurray 1991, p. 210)

The study revealed that one of the most notable characteristics of the expert community health nurse is her or his superior communication skills. Experts in the study spent a large proportion of time listening, clarifying and using the 'self' therapeutically, in a facilitative capacity. One expert nurse explained that she has no set role, but is able to adapt to how she 'reads' the need once she enters the home. This therapeutic and situationally circumscribed role allows her to attend consciously to the client, interact as a partner in self-care and assess both the problems that are being discussed and the dynamics of the interaction so that she can judge the situation, set priorities for action and enable needs to be met. This is exemplified in Case 6.1 'Working with a multiproblem family' (p. 130).

One of the ways in which superior communication skills was manifest in the study group was in the prominence of using a culturally sensitive approach, particularly in such places as high school settings. Instead of asking a student direct questions about his or her family,the nurse would most often begin the line of questioning with something like 'And who lives at your house?', acknowledging the diversity of family structures in the various communities. Nurses' comments during their client interviews were also important. Comments which reflected the integration of what was observed ('You seem upset'), what was heard ('You're concerned about'), and the context ('I suppose it doesn't help being in the suburbs with no transportation') served as triggers which stimulated the client to provide further information (McMurray 1992a).

Several nurses explained the importance of effective communication strategies in the context of reassuring clients. Most community health nurses believe in the importance of reassuring parents that they are doing a good job with their children, yet some of the experts who participated in the study suggested that the timing of reassurance must be chosen carefully. One nurse explained this as learning from experience to reassure as a means of providing accurate feedback at the appropriate time rather than to reassure as a matter of course, as if to pacify the client. The latter, according to one expert, runs the risk of prematurely closing off the conversation and may even inhibit the client or parent in developing new or more satisfying approaches to child rearing.

Kasch (1986a, 1986b) suggests that the nurse must become a communication strategist by interpretively assessing the perspectives and constraints of others; an essential component of competent nursing action which he calls 'relational competence' (Kasch 1986a, p. 45). According to this author, nurses are able to empower clients for self-care by establishing collaborative provider-client relationships which requires 'interaction management: the ability to start, maintain and regulate conversations in a way that encourages the elicitation and elaboration of the patient's perspective' (Kasch 1986b, p. 46).

Community health nurses who participated in the study of expertise demonstrated relational competence in a wide variety of client encounters.

Perhaps this competency is more easily developed in the community than in acute care settings, because of the continuing nature of the nurse-client relationship. In many cases observed, nurses set priorities and plans for care which were tempered by a sense of time, a luxury which is unique to community health nursing. As one school health nurse declared: 'You need to be very patient. You can sit on something for a month or two until it all comes together. They're not medical emergencies. They're social emergencies, but not immediately life threatening. You need to judge the difference between "I'm going to kill myself" and "I'm **going** to kill myself"' (McMurray 1991, p. 202).

Child health nurses also mentioned this sense of time. One nurse reflected on the case of a young mother having difficulty adjusting after the birth of her child as follows: 'She repeatedly comes to me with a variety of problems, yet when it comes time for dealing with them, "roadblocks" my attempts to help. With each encounter I look at alternatives as to why she is doing this, gathering cues, and knowing that in time I will get to the real problem' (McMurray 1991, p. 202).

This sense of time and the opportunity to follow up on nursing interventions is an aspect which attracts many nurses to practise with families in the community where the nurse's personal resourcefulness pays such large dividends. In one nurse's words: 'You always have to be trying and thinking laterally or creatively because things are always changing' (McMurray 1991, p. 209). This seemingly simplistic statement captures the essence of community health nursing. It is an opportunity for personal and professional growth in the process of helping people to help themselves. A final vignette is presented here in an attempt to encapsulate the level of sophistication in exemplary community health nursing practice.

Case 6.4: Exemplary school health nursing practice

A school health nurse arrived for her weekly visit to the local primary school, stopping by the teachers' lunch room to see whether any of their students were in need of her services. As her informal discussion got under way, a football came through the window and all the teachers exclaimed: 'Harry!' (a pseudonym). He was immediately described as a behaviour problem, with individual teachers lending substance to the label with their own examples, one of which involved glue sniffing with some of his other black friends. The principal decided to turn Harry over to the nurse to solve his problems. The nurse took him to a quiet place and asked him to explain why he thought he had been sent to her. She listened to his perception of the problem (the football incident), asking him to clarify his feelings about his teachers, his friends and the school as these topics had arisen in the conversation. Once he was finished talking and she had gathered a great deal of information, she confronted him with the real issue: that he had been seen sniffing glue. She did not wait for him to excuse his behaviour, but began slowly and calmly to remind him of what he had just told her. She reflected back to him a picture of a boy who felt discriminated against, explaining that the problem lay with those who discriminated, not with him. She portrayed an athlete who was much better at football than his glue-sniffing friends, and praised him on his goal to enter the upcoming field day and to eventually be the first of his large family to make it into (and through) high school. At no time did she level any accusations, but rather, asked him if he could see the incompatibility in the two images of the boy sniffing glue (weakness) and the other who was destined for success (strength). The most salient features of the interaction were the nurse's ability to listen, to be non-judgemental, to impart a caring image, to understand the situation in terms of his goals and social environment, and to communicate her message at the boy's level of understanding. The nurse's interaction with the boy was aimed at empowering him to make his own choices.

(McMurray 1991, pp. 207-208)

When asked to reflect on the encounter and her level of sensitivity, the nurse described it as one where you learn to understand people in the context of their family and their culture by listening. She reported that she has learned to seek students' opinions, to listen to them and take notice of them. She predicted very decisively that, in collaborating to nurture and reinforce the boy's strengths, she and the school team could effect a positive outcome for him and, perhaps, for others in his family. Her approach demonstrates equity, access, empowerment, cultural sensitivity and self-determinism; the goals of primary health care put into practice. The encounter illustrates the characteristics of an expert which operate synchronously (Fig. 6.5).

1. Knowledge of individual functioning and the capacity for self-care, family dynamics, patterns of human response in health and illness and the social conditions which precipitate conditions, abilities and responses
2. Clinical judgement, the ability to get right to the problem
3. Client-centred empathy, the ability to understand the perspective of the client

4. Self-confidence in her or his perceptions, judgements and intervention strategies
5. Holistic understanding of the individual and family in the context of culture and community
6. Appropriate communication (relational competence).

(McMurray 1991, p. 174)

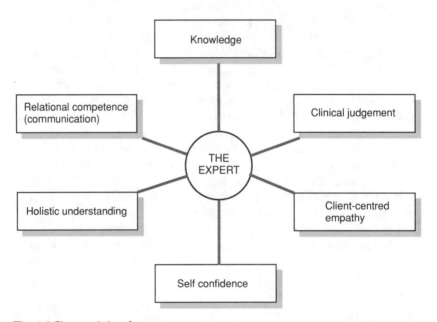

Fig. 6.5 Characteristics of an expert.

BECOMING AN EXPERT COMMUNITY HEALTH NURSE

Benner (1984) suggests that the development of expertise follows a five-stage model of skills acquisition first described by Dreyfus and Dreyfus (1986). She explains that nurses, like other learners, may progress in stages from novice to advanced beginner, competent, proficient to expert as illustrated in Table 6.1.

According to the model, the expert is distinguished by her or his intuitive grasp and deep understanding of a situation, and the tendency to base actions or interventions on this type of understanding rather than on an analysis of constituent elements. Experience plays an essential role in the process of acquiring this level of understanding. Kolodner (1984) explains that experience serves to turn unrelated facts into expert knowledge through two processes. First, knowledge is built up incrementally as facts become integrated through occurrence in the same types of episodes. Second, reasoning processes are refined, and as a result of noticing failures and

Table 6.1   Dreyfus model of skill acquisition

Stage 1:	Novice—The novice acquires rules for determining actions based upon objectively defined elements and without consideration of the overall situation.
Stage 2:	Advanced Beginner—Through practical experience in meaningful situations the advanced beginner begins to identify aspects of a situation.
Stage 3:	Competent—With increasing experience, actions are seen in terms of long-term goals or plans, based on conscious, abstract, analytic contemplation of problems.
Stage 4:	Proficient—Sophisticated analysis allows the proficient person to see situations as a whole.
Stage 5:	Expert—There is no longer a reliance on analytic principles; skills have become a part of the expert. A deep situational understanding allows one to focus on the accurate region of a problem without wasteful consideration of alternatives.

(Dreyfus & Dreyfus 1986)

successes, and differences and similarities between cases, the ability to deal with exceptional or novel cases is derived. Experience guides the reasoning process by the way it is organized in long term memory, either reinforcing successful past performance or, in the case of failures, providing a basis for guiding changes to the memory organization and consequently to the reasoning processes themselves. However, not all experienced nurses become experts. Expertise seems to develop from a combination of personal factors (for example, being a motivated, receptive and confident individual) being exposed to effective role models, having life experiences which one is able to integrate with professional experiences (for example, parenting and/or travel) and educational opportunities which stimulate both perceptual and analytic abilities (see Fig. 6.6).

Although the accrual of experiences cannot always be controlled, there would appear to be many and varied opportunities for developing expertise in community health nursing by virtue of the nature of practice. Nurses practising in home visiting are provided with a wide variety of families, circumstances and health related issues to use as a frame of reference for future cases. In the school setting, the nurse is confronted with a broad spectrum of child and adolescent issues, each of which is embedded in its own individual social and familial contexts. Child health nurses, like other community health nurses, are exposed to family issues which reflect not only changing family configurations but evolving societal attitudes and values. In occupational health settings, nurses are exposed to the special issues surrounding health maintenance in the world of work. Community health nursing thus provides unique and varied experiences. It provides the template for developing receptivity, the opportunity to capitalize on personal and previous professional experiences, a forum for consolidating educational experiences and most importantly, time to reflect upon practice issues, memories and future plans. It is fertile ground for the development of expertise.

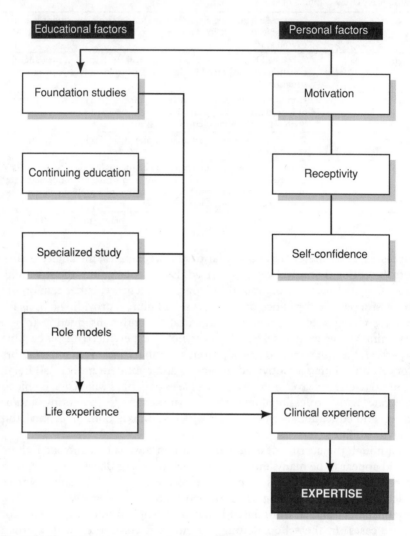

Fig. 6.6 The development of expertise (From McMurray 1992a).

SUMMARY

This chapter has provided a mere glimpse into an intriguing and vital aspect of community health nursing: nursing the family. A community's social functioning, and therefore the social dimension of community health, is dependent upon the integrity of the family unit. As the link between individuals and society, the family transmits attitudes and values from the family to society and reciprocally, from society to the family.

It is becoming increasingly important for the community health nurse to understand the richness of family nursing with all its complexities, as the practice activities of many nurses primarily revolve around the family. The previous discussion has attempted to provide a general overview of theoretical perspectives of the family and to examine the process of assessing and caring for families. Family nursing may be practised by using the process-oriented approach discussed in Chapter 4; however expert nurses also draw upon intuitive judgements in planning nursing care strategies for the family and community. Several examples of this type of approach to practice were presented in this chapter to provide a window on expertise in community health nursing. These examples attempted to illustrate how expert nurses work in partnership with families in the community to facilitate improved health status. Finally, a model for the development of expertise in community health nursing was presented. The section to follow extends the discussion of family nursing to a more generalized exploration of the processes of health education and health promotion and to the need and methods of researching *all* areas of community health nursing practice.

Study exercises

1. All community health nursing is family nursing. Discuss.
2. Conduct an assessment on a family in your community using Friedman's family health assessment form.
3. What would you anticipate as the two most important issues facing a parent who is leaving the home as a result of separation or divorce?
4. How does the grieving process of a parent whose child has died differ from that of one who has been denied custody? What are the implications for nurses?
5. What resources would prove most helpful to a family caring for an 83-year-old frail aunt?
6. Analyze the concept of empathy. How important do you think empathy is in developing relational competence? Explain.
7. Is it possible to use an holistic approach for assessing all cultures? What are some of the culture-specific issues that must be considered in the assessment process?
8. Give three examples of reassuring comments to parents and provide a brief description of a situation where each would be appropriate and three where each would be inappropriate.

REFERENCES

Amato P 1987 Children in Australian families: the growth of competence. Australian Institute of Family Studies, Melbourne and Prentice-Hall, Sydney
Anderson J 1990 Home care management in chronic illness and the self-care movement: an analysis of ideologies and economic processes influencing policy decisions. Advances in Nursing Science 12(2):71-83

Benner P 1984 From novice to expert: excellence and power in clinical nursing practice. Addison-Wesley, Menlo Park

Benner P, Tanner C 1987 How expert nurses use intuition. American Journal of Nursing 87(1):23-31

Berne A, Dato C, Mason D, Rafferty M 1992 A nursing model for addressing the health needs of homeless families. In: Saucier K (ed) Perspectives in family and community health. C V Mosby, St Louis, pp 369-377

Burns A 1981 Divorce and the children. Australian Journal of Sex, Marriage & Family 2:17-26

Butrin J (1992) Cultural diversity in the nurse-client encounter. Clinical Nursing Research 1(3):238-251

Butterfield P 1992 Thinking upstream: nurturing a conceptual understanding of the societal context of health behaviour. In: Saucier K (ed) Perspectives in family and community health. C V Mosby, St Louis, pp 66-71

Carneiro C 1985 Cultural diversity and the family. In: Jarvis L (ed) Community health nursing: keeping the public healthy, 2nd edn. F A Davis, Philadelphia, pp 205-228

Carey R 1992 How values affect the mutual goal setting process with multiproblem families. In: Saucier K (ed) Perspectives in family and community health. C V Mosby, St Louis, pp 320-325

Carter E, McGoldrick M 1980 The family life cycle: a framework for family therapy. Gardner Press, New York

Dreyfus H, Dreyfus S 1986 Mind over machine: the power of human intuition and expertise in the era of the computer. The Free Press, New York

Duffy M 1992 Strategies for change: the one parent family. In: Saucier K (ed) Perspectives in family and community health. C V Mosby, St Louis, pp 326-333

Duvall E 1977 Marriage and family relationships, 5th edn. Lippincott, Philadelphia

Eastman M 1989 Family: the vital factor. Collins Dove, Melbourne

Edgar D 1991 Families and the social reconstruction of marriage and parenthood in Australia. In: Batten R, Weeks W, Wilson J (eds) Issues facing Australian families. Longman Cheshire, Melbourne, pp 3-19

Friedman M 1986 Family nursing: theory and assessment, 2nd edn. Appleton-Century-Crofts, Norwalk

Furstenberg F, Nord C 1985 Parenting apart: patterns of child rearing after marital disruption. Journal of Marriage and the Family 48 (May):438-447

Glasser M, Prohaska T, Roska J 1992 The role of the family in medical care-seeking decisions of older adults. Family Community Health 15(2):59-70

Halpern R 1992 Poverty and early childhood parenting: toward a framework for intervention. In: Saucier K (ed) Perspectives in family and community health. C V Mosby, St Louis, pp 357-368

Hetherington E, Cox M, Cox R 1977 The aftermath of divorce. In: Stevens J, Matthews M (eds) Mother-child father-child relationships. National Association for the Education of Young Children, Washington

Institute for the Development of Educational Activities and National Association of Elementary School Principals 1980 The most significant minority: one parent children in the schools

Johnson R 1988 Family developmental theories. In: Stanhope M, Lancaster J (eds) Community health nursing: process and practice for promoting health, 2nd edn. C V Mosby, St Louis, pp 352-370

Johnson J 1991 Learning to live again: the process of adjustment following a heart attack. In: Morse J, Johnson J (eds) The illness experience: dimensions of suffering. Sage, Newbury Park pp 13-88

Kasch C 1986a Establishing a collaborative nurse-patient relationship: a distinct focus of nursing action in primary care. Image: The Journal of Nursing Scholarship 18(2):226-230

Kasch C 1986b Toward a theory of nursing action: skills and competency in nurse-patient interaction. Nursing Research 35(4):226-230

Kolodner J 1984 Towards an understanding of the role of experience in the evolution from novice to expert. In: Langlotz C, Shortliffe E (eds) Developments in expert systems. Academic Press, London

Leininger M 1978 Transcultural nursing concepts, theories and practices. Wiley, New York

Loveland-Cherry C 1992 Issues in family health promotion. In: Stanhope M, Lancaster J (eds) Community health nursing: process and practice for promoting health, 3rd edn. Mosby, St Louis, pp 470-483

Lynch I, Tiedje L 1991 Working with multiproblem families: an intervention model for community health nurses. Public Health Nursing 8(3):147-153

McCaughey J 1987 A bit of a struggle: coping with family life in Australia, McPhee Gribble, Melbourne

McMurray A 1991 Expertise in community health nursing. Unpublished doctoral thesis, Department of Education, The University of Western Australia, Perth

McMurray 1992a Expertise in community health nursing. Journal of Community Health Nursing 9(2):65-75

McMurray A 1992b Influences on parent-child relationships in non-custodial mothers. Australian Journal of Marriage & Family 13(3):138-147

Minuchin S 1974 Families and family therapy. Harvard University Press, Cambridge

Minuchin S 1984 Family kaleidoscope. Harvard University Press, Cambridge

Moccia P, Mason D 1986 Poverty trends: implications for nursing. Nursing Outlook 34(1):20

O'Neill C, Sorensen E 1991 Home care of the elderly: a family perspective. Advances in Nursing Science 13(4):28-37

Pease B, Wilson J 1991 Men in families. In: Batten R, Weeks W, Wilson J (eds) Issues facing Australian families, Longman Cheshire, Melbourne, pp 54-64

Pratt L 1976 Family structure and effective health behaviour. Houghton Mifflin, Boston

Pyles S, Stern P 1983 Discovery of nursing gestalt in critical care nursing: the importance of the gray gorilla syndrome. Image: The Journal of Nursing Scholarship 15(2):51-57

Rew L 1988 Intuition in decision making. Image: The Journal of Nursing Scholarship 20(3):150-153

Satir V 1967 Conjoint family therapy. Science & Behavior Books, Palo Alto

Schon D 1983 The reflective practitioner. Basic Books, New York

Turner-Henson A, Holaday B, Swan J 1992 When parenting becomes care giving: caring for the chronically ill child. Family Community Health 15(2):19-30

Twinn S 1991 Conflicting paradigms of health visiting: a continuing debate for professional practice. Journal of Advanced Nursing 16:966-973

Wallerstein J, Kelly J 1980 Surviving the breakup: how children and parents cope with divorce, Grant McIntyre, London

Watson P 1992 Family issues in rehabilitation, Holistic Nursing Practice 6(2):51-59

Weitzman L 1986 The divorce revolution: the unexpected social and economic consequences for women and children in America. The Free Press, New York

Wilson S 1992 The family as care givers: hospice home care. Family Community Health 15(2):71-80

Wright L, Leahey M 1984 Nurses and families: a guide to family assessment and intervention. F A Davis, Philadelphia

Wright L, Leahey M 1987 Families & chronic illness. Springhouse Corp, Pennsylvania

PART 4

Health education, health promotion and research

INTRODUCTION

The pivotal process of community health nursing is concerned with promoting and maintaining the health of community members, either as individuals, families or groups defined by culture or interest. In many cases, this involves becoming an agent of change and a partner in health care. In order to function effectively in this role, the community health nurse must base his or her practice on a sound theoretical basis which includes, but is not limited to, the collective body of knowledge advanced by theorists, such as was discussed in Chapter 3. In order to provide informed choices for communities, the nurse must also adopt a research perspective, either by actively challenging existing knowledge through participation in the research process, or by incorporating current research findings into practice. This section presents a discussion of the techniques and strategies for educating and promoting health in the community in Chapter 7, then describes the process of researching issues relevant to community health nursing in Chapter 8. It is expected that as a critical mass of knowledge accumulates through research, the processes of promoting and maintaining health in communities will be challenged, refuted, validated or revised in a way that will be beneficial to communities as well as those who care for them.

Content: Part 4

7. Health education and health promotion

Health education
Health promotion
   The Healthy Cities Project
Health promotion approaches
   Group approaches to health promotion
   Group approaches to health education
   The teacher-facilitator
   Steps in the teaching-facilitating process
The role of the nurse in health education and promotion

8. The research process

Why research?
The process of research
Questions for investigation
   Accessibility of health care
   Community involvement
   Appropriate technology
   Multisectoral approach
Methods for community health nursing research
Epidemiology
   The epidemiological triad model
   The person-place-time model
   The web of causation model
   Epidemiological measures
     Descriptive measures
     Analytic measures
   Study design
   Epidemiology in community health nursing

7. Health education and health promotion

A large part of community health nursing practice revolves around helping people change. In some cases this is a matter of working with individuals or groups to help people maximize strengths and resources, or to understand where change would be helpful in achieving higher levels of health or wellness. In this respect, the nurse is said to function as a 'change agent', one who potentiates or facilitates change. As an agent of change, the nurse is usually engaged in health education, health promotion or both. As these two terms are often used interchangeably, some definitions follow.

HEALTH EDUCATION

Health education, according to Green and Kreuter (1991), is planned educational intervention aimed primarily at the voluntary actions people can take on their own (individually or collectively) as citizens looking after their own health or as decision-makers looking after the health of others and the common good of the community.

HEALTH PROMOTION

Health promotion encompasses health education and is aimed at 'the complementary social and political actions that will facilitate the necessary organizational, economic and other environmental supports for the conversion of individual actions into health enhancement and quality of life gains' (Green & Kreuter 1991, p. 14). Health promotion thus extends health education to the primary health care focus on social and political action in the expectation that people will be able to lobby for the social changes which provide the *opportunities* as well as the education to improve their health status (Milio 1981).

As mentioned in Chapter 1, the goals of community health promotion strategies are to:

- build healthy public policies
- create supportive environments
- strengthen community action
- develop personal skills
- reorient health services.

(Ottawa Charter for Health Promotion 1986)

Green and Kreuter (1991) suggest that these goals can be met if health promotion strategies are based on a systematic approach which begins with a community educational diagnosis which is multidimensional and situationally specific. Educational needs are identified from a thorough individual, group or community assessment and validated with the client(s) to ensure relevance. Such needs may be as simple as a new parent's need for instruction on infant feeding, or as complex as a community-identified need for employment retraining programs. Green and Kreuter (1991) offer the Precede-Proceed model as a guide to health promotion planning and evaluation (see Fig. 7.1).

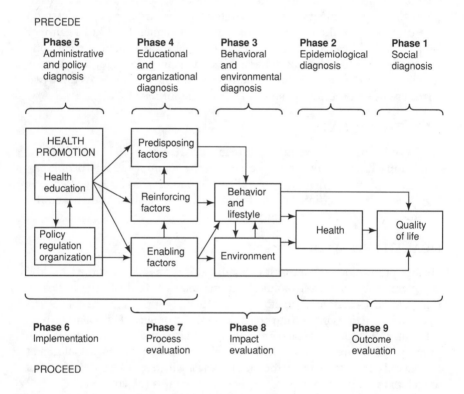

Fig. 7.1 The PRECEDE-PROCEED model for health promotion planning and evaluation (From Green & Kreuter 1991).

Green and Kreuter (1991) explain that the model is best used if the change agent begins with the final consequences (quality of life) then works back deductively to the original causes. This involves nine phases as follows:

Phase 1: Social diagnosis

The process begins with an assessment of a community's needs and aspirations. This can best be accomplished by involving the community in defining what health related outcomes they would like to achieve. These outcomes take the form of social indicators, and include such variables as level of personal achievement, crime, crowding, discrimination and unemployment.

Phase 2: Epidemiological diagnosis

During this phase, the specific health goals or problems that may contribute to the social goals or problems noted in Phase 1 are identified and ranked. This includes assessing such vital indicators as morbidity, mortality, disability, and fertility, and identifying dimensions of each (incidence, prevalence, intensity).

Phase 3: Behavioural and environmental diagnosis

At this stage the specific health related behavioural and environmental factors which impact on the health problems targeted for action are identified and ranked. Behavioural indicators include for example, compliance, consumption patterns, coping, preventive actions, and self-care. Dimensions of these behavioural factors include frequency, persistence, promptness, quality and range. Indicators from the economic, physical, services and social environment are also ranked with their dimensions of access, affordability and equity. A Phase 3 diagnosis would therefore constitute specific dimensions of particular indicators, such as the frequency (dimension) of alcohol consumption among middle-age males (behavioural indicator) or the access (dimension) to child care for working single mothers (environmental indicator).

Phase 4: Educational and organizational diagnosis

At this stage, the predisposing, reinforcing and enabling factors which would be most likely to bring about behavioural and environmental change are identified and prioritized. Predisposing factors include a person or group's knowledge, attitudes, values and perceptions that facilitate or hinder motivation for change. For example, believing that health can be affected by lifestyle, maintaining an attitude of self-confidence in caring for oneself, and valuing life itself would be considered positive predisposing factors. Reinforcing factors include the attitudes and behaviours of others (health professionals, peers, parents, employers) which are likely to reinforce any behaviour change. Enabling factors are those skills (self-awareness), resources (employment), or barriers (poverty) that can help or hinder the desired changes as well as environmental changes.

Phase 5: Administrative and policy diagnosis

Organizational and administrative capabilities and resources are assessed at this stage. The assessment concludes with selecting the right level and combination of methods and strategies (individual, group and/or mass media), the deployment of intervention staff, and the launching of the community organization or organizational development process. For example, a much more energetic and well resourced AIDS prevention campaign would be launched when a political party has just been voted in on a program of social reforms, than during a period of voter preoccupation with employment, such as occurs during a recession.

Phase 6: Implementation

This phase represents the culmination of each of the previous phases. Implementation should be as comprehensive as possible, given the information which surfaces from the diagnostic exercises. Hawe et al (1992) use the example of child abuse in a new housing estate to illustrate the interplay of risk factors. Once a diagnosis of risk factors has been made, a multi-stage and/or multifactorial plan may be implemented which targets as many of these factors (stress, a lack of child care, low social support, poor parenting skills and a lack of play or recreation facilities) as possible. The plan must then be packaged in such a way as to be acceptable to the community. This is best accomplished through social marketing; that is, developing the right *product* backed by the right *promotion* and put in the right *place* at the right *price* (Kotler 1975). For health education and promotion, the product is the program. To be marketed successfully, it must be developed for the needs and interests of the target population. Promotion strategies aim to make the program visible and attractive. Place relates to the means and logistics of making the program acceptable, while cost may include the money, time, or energy required to deliver the program (Dignan & Carr 1987).

Phases 7, 8, 9: Evaluation

Evaluation is an integral and continuous part of the entire diagnostic process. The criteria for evaluation are derived from the educational objectives. The extent to which these objectives are met represents process evaluation (Hawe et al 1992). Objects of the evaluative process for Phases 7 and 8 thus include measures of quality of life; health status indicators; behavioural and environmental factors, predisposing, reinforcing and enabling factors; intervention activities; methods of delivery; changes in policies, regulations, or organizations; level of staff expertise; and quality of performance: and educational materials. The overall outcome evaluation (Phase 9) represents a measure of the extent to which the global objectives were met (impact evaluation) and whether or not the program goal was met (outcome evaluation). Phase 9 thus compares the 'object of interest against a standard of acceptability' (Green & Kreuter 1991, p. 217).

Many successful health promotion campaigns have been undertaken in Australia, and although they have not always been described in terms of the Precede-Proceed model, they have included the principles suggested by Green and Kreuter and the Ottawa Charter for Health Promotion. For example, the North Coast Healthy Lifestyle Program which began in 1979 (Egger et al 1983) adopted a multidimensional, situationally specific approach to promoting the health of a community (Lismore) on the North Coast of New South Wales (NSW). The program (which this author was involved in at the time) used a variety of strategies to achieve change in individual behaviour and in community systems and structures (Esler-McMurray 1980, Egger et al 1990). First, the NSW Health Commission was lobbied to initiate healthy public policies which would result in funding for the campaign. The next step was aimed at creating a supportive environment. The media (radio, TV, newspaper) was used extensively and creatively to frame health education messages so that the average community resident could identify with them. In other words, images portrayed typical people rather than glamorous role models. The nurse, as part of the interdisciplinary team, participated in the preparation of the media messages. Next, all general practitioners in the area were visited by the nurse involved to ensure their support for the program and to keep them abreast of each phase of the campaign. The local butchers were contacted to explain that the campaign was going to include urging people to trim the fat from their meat and to ask for their support. Chemists were also contacted to involve them in an aspect of the campaign which was aimed at encouraging community residents to have their medications checked. The local teachers were also involved at each step so that they could anticipate the physical fitness campaign and reinforce the messages being sent out to their students via the media.

The strategy selected to strengthen community action was to employ a 'pull' rather than a 'push' model to allow many community groups to have input into the program and to choose freely the extent of their involvement. As a result, various groups such as the Country Women's Association (CWA) and the Returned Serviceman's League (RSL) became involved, some members volunteering to provide information to community residents, others ensuring access to various venues for parts of the program. The butchers became very involved with the campaign, providing advice on low fat cuts of meat. Their zeal was encouraged when each had a turn being photographed for the local paper 'trimming the meat'. In effect, they accepted a degree of ownership with the campaign, as did the chemists, who were also featured in the local paper as they provided advice to people on 'pill day', a designated day each month when the public was invited to bring their medications in for identification or advice.

An anti-hypertension program was also instituted, which involved an educational component as well as community screening by the nurse. This program attempted to help people develop personal skills for identifying and coping with high blood pressure and related health factors. Other aspects of the campaign aimed at developing personal skills included smoking cessation, nutrition awareness, physical fitness, stress management and healthy ageing. Each of these aspects used a re-oriented health service to get to the people. A shop front 'Healthy Lifestyle Shop' offered a variety of educational and diagnostic services in a very accessible part of the shopping area. Included were videotapes on health topics, quit smoking kits, cooking demonstrations, fitness testing, and blood pressure pamphlets. This community-based health promotion service set an example for several other shop fronts for health promotion in Adelaide, Perth, Darwin, Hobart and Sydney (Egger et al 1990).

This type of health promotion approach which uses community organization has also been used in a variety of other places including Finland (McAlister et al 1981), the USA (Maccoby & Solomon 1981, Lasater et al 1988), and Wales (Nutbeam & Catford 1987). Each program can lay claim to immediate indicators of improved health, however, the most important and enduring outcome in each case is the influence on community attitudes toward health issues which ultimately result in behavioural and structural changes. One would expect such programs to proliferate in an ideal world; however, in this era of economic rationalism comprehensive health promotion campaigns are considered too costly and have been easily replaced by short term programs which have more immediate outcomes. One exception is the Healthy Cities Project, an initiative of the WHO.

The Healthy Cities Project

The rationale of the Healthy Cities Project lies in the recognition of social health as a vital component of new public health practice in industrialized cities (Baum & Brown 1989) and the 'realization that more than half of the world's population lives in cities, where the problems are most concentrated and the resources are most plentiful' (Flynn 1992, p. 13). This represents a shift away from the individual focus of early health promotion campaigns to the conditions of living which set the level of risk for health or illness. English and Hicks (1992) suggest that the Healthy Cities concept acknowledges the importance of understanding a community's political processes and the conflicts inherent in human interaction. Community health nurses involved in such projects will be able to make use of their 'skills in community development, coalition building, networking, advocacy, mutual support group facilitation, the facilitation of empowerment, and the use of the media' (English & Hicks 1992, p. 64).

The idea of the city as the social unit through which to address health promotion strategies emerged from a meeting of representatives from 17 European cities in Lisbon in 1986 and was based on the premise that the first responsibility of a city is to promote the health of its residents (Brown 1992). The WHO acted as a facilitator at the international level to assist a network of cities around the world to 'extrapolate health promotion activities, especially multisectoral action and community participation, to the local level, (McPherson 1992, p. 124). Participants at the Lisbon meeting defined a healthy city as one in which:

- 'health is a social rather than a medical matter;
- health is the responsibility of all city services;
- health should be monitored by physical, social aesthetic and environmental indicators of well being;
- health is an outcome of collaboration between community members, planners and providers of public and private sector services;
- the city should be a cradle of good health and not merely a survival unit.'

(Baum & Brown 1989, p. 141).

The Healthy Cities initiative is now a world wide movement with over 400 cities participating in 17 national networks, each committed to the goal of encouraging local government involvement in health promotion (Flynn 1992). In 1986, three Australian cities, Canberra (ACT), Illawarra (NSW) and Noarlunga (SA) established Healthy Cities initiatives as a pilot project under the auspices of the Australian Community Health Association. Since that time these pilot cities have been joined by a fourth, the Nganampa Health Council, which provides health services for the Aboriginal people living on the Pitjantjatjara lands in Central Australia, and other Healthy Cities projects are being planned for Western Australia, Tasmania, Queensland, South Australia and New South Wales (Baum et al 1992). Each city has a team of health professionals, representatives of recreation, police, social services, voluntary organizations, young and older people to develop and test the applicability of intersectoral collaboration in meeting the objectives of the Ottawa Charter for Health Promotion (Baum & Brown 1989). Most cities embarking on Healthy Cities initiatives begin by undertaking specific projects which encourage commitment to the approach, demonstrate its effectiveness and promote the ideas of co-operation and better health at the local level. Healthy Cities initiatives have included such things as environmental clean-ups, tree-planting schemes, health expos, and road safety campaigns (Healthy Cities Australia 1991). The Healthy Cities network thus provides a vehicle for primary health care in Australia as well as in other industrialized Western countries. Ongoing evaluation and monitoring of the projects will determine future developments in other cities.

HEALTH PROMOTION APPROACHES

Health promotion programs can be conducted using an individual, group or mass media approach. In the past, health promotion occurred on a one-to-one basis, in the home (mother to child) or in health care settings (physician, child health nurse or midwife to patient). In today's society, individual approaches are often too costly as compared to the number of people who may be reached through mass media campaigns. Despite the advantages of one-to-one communication, many health promotion programs target the group, often to complement individualized strategies. According to Egger et al (1990, p. 50) group techniques offer 'an intermediary between one-to-one approaches and wider community appeals through media and whole community approaches'.

Group approaches to health promotion

For a variety of reasons, including resource limitations, many health promotion campaigns focus on a particular group. In some situations, in order to effect the desired change in one group, another group whose behaviour affects the target group must also be targeted (Hawe et al 1992). For example, parents, or teachers are often included in strategies to bring about change in children or adolescents. Some campaigns target those at risk for particular conditions such as cervical cancer (Hirst et al 1990), breast cancer (Turnbull et al 1991), cardiovascular disease (James et al 1989, 1990), AIDS (Connell et al 1991), or alcohol related problems (Health Department of Western Australia 1988). In order to devise programs that are appropriate for the group at risk, research must be undertaken into all phases of health promotion planning, particularly during the diagnostic stage. One example of how Green and Kreuter's (1991) five phases of educational diagnosis can be used to guide health promotion is described below in using the Health Department of Western Australia's (HDWA) 'Drinksafe' program as a basis for health promotion on a university campus.

As part of a practicum exercise, nursing students at Edith Cowan University developed a health promotion program targeting drinking behaviour in 18–25-year-old university students.

Phase 1: Social diagnosis

From the literature and HDWA statistics the students identified increased absenteeism, decreased worker productivity and domestic violence (all related to alcohol use) as the major social implications of alcohol misuse in the general community. Visible social effects in the university community included poor attendance at classes, falling grades and difficulties with interpersonal relationships.

Phase 2: Epidemiological diagnosis

In this second phase, the students discovered that in 1991, 5% of deaths in Western Australia were attributable to alcohol. In 1988, over 36 000 bed days for men and over 21 000 bed days for women were attributable to alcohol related disease (Holman 1991). The data did not reveal whether any of these were students.

Phase 3: Behavioural and environmental diagnosis

The next phase revealed a high prevalence of 18–25-year-olds regularly drinking alcohol and a high incidence of 18–25-year-olds booked by the police for drink driving.

Phase 4: Educational and organizational diagnosis

Predisposing factors. Through peer discussions, the students suspected that there may be a lack of knowledge about safe drinking levels among 18-25-year-olds, and that many of this target group held the attitude or belief that 'getting caught drink driving won't happen to me'. Furthermore, the students hoped to overcome any incorrect perceptions of the amount of alcohol required to get drunk. They also considered the various beliefs related to alcohol use, such as cultural beliefs in some households that alcohol with meals is beneficial.

Reinforcing factors. The factors familiar to the students which sustain drinking behaviour were identified as peer approval and, in some cases, parent approval, and the ever presence of alcohol in the media.

Enabling factors. The students identified the enabling factors as the availability of alcohol, the low cost of alcohol, the proliferation of pub promotions offering free drinks and, related to the drink driving factor, a lack of public transport.

Phase 5: Administrative and policy diagnosis

In order to mount an effective campaign, the students looked into the policies which would impact on drinking behaviour. These included legislation for safe driving (0.05 blood alcohol limit) and the introduction of Random Breath Testing (RBT), both of which were designed to act as deterrents to overuse of alcohol.

The Drinksafe campaign in the university community

The students organizing the campaign decided to introduce the following health education strategies:

1. Individual. Information booklets on safe drinking levels were distributed throughout the campus. These were readily available through the state Drinksafe campaign. In the primary health care clinic (a demonstration clinic in the school of nursing) the students also offered individualized computer assessment of alcohol use to all students and staff wishing to take part. This was also promoted throughout the campus.

2. Group. The students conducted an educational seminar on drink driving. Educational videotapes on alcohol related issues were shown in the campus cafeteria as well as in the primary health care clinic.

3. Mass media. Posters and pamphlets supplied by the state Drinksafe campaign were displayed in campus libraries and other places (such as pubs) where 18-25-year-olds tend to gather.

The goal of the program was to bring about a reduction in morbidity and mortality associated with alcohol intake in 18-25 year olds. Specific program objectives included:

Educational objectives. After some discussion, the students running the campaign decided that realistic expectations for change six months after implementation of the program would include the following:

- 80% of 18-25-year-olds on campus would be able to state the safe drinking limits
- 80% of liquor outlets in the immediate community surrounding the campus would provide low alcohol beer
- 80% of 18-25-year-old students at the university would receive further information about alcohol use.

Behavioural objective. The students decided that it would also be realistic to expect that six months after implementation of the program there would be a 20% reduction in the number of 18-25-year-old university students in the community booked for drink driving.

The students suggested that these objectives be evaluated at a period of six months following the program's implementation with the evaluation results used as the basis for revision or renewal of the program. Because this group of students had to move on from the project within six months, they were unable to monitor the evaluation through to its conclusion; however, their expectation was that the campus-wide program would at least parallel the success of the state Drinksafe program. According to the HDWA (1988), surveys conducted 18 months after the launch of the Drinksafe program indicated that there had been a decrease in the percentage of men and women who exceed the limits of drinking alcohol recommended by the National Health and Medical Research Council in any week. These surveys also indicated a reduction in the average number of days on which people drink alcohol, and other surveys suggested that Western Australian drinkers are becoming better informed about the health risks of drinking too much alcohol, lending credence to the campaign strategies (Clarke & Knowles 1990).

Research into health promotion issues informs the process of promoting health as well as preventing illness and injury in the community by providing diagnostic evidence which can ultimately lead to the development of public policies (Wintemute 1992). For example, Australian research such as Adelson et al's (1992) study of the type of women who attend screening mammography assists the process of social diagnosis for this issue. Burnley's (1991) study of stomach cancer mortality in NSW and Sydney provides information from which to make an epidemiological diagnosis. Behavioural and environmental diagnoses are clarified by studies such as Donnelly et al's (1992) research into trends in drug prevalence among secondary school students. Educational and organizational factors have been explored by Hall et al (1992) who studied the public perception of the risks and benefits of alcohol, and by the Borland et al (1992) study of smoking prevalence following a total workplace smoking ban. However, despite a growing body of literature, there have been very few studies which address the issue of empowerment, which lies at the heart of the Ottawa Charter for Health

Promotion (Raeburn & Beaglehole 1989). In order to devise health promotion strategies that are equitable, accessible, and self-determined, research studies must explore the issues which impact on community and group participation to identify the circumstances under which communities and groups within those communities become empowered (Wallerstein 1992).

Group approaches to health education

Although health education is often conducted on an individual basis, a considerable proportion of teaching occurs in groups. For the nurse or other health professional planning health education presentations, the decision must be made whether to conduct individual or group sessions. There are times when each is appropriate. Confidentiality is more easily maintained in a one-to-one situation. In addition, it is easier to determine an individual learner's motivation, readiness to learn, and knowledge level. On the other hand, group teaching is an economical way to present material to many learners. Group learners are also advantaged by a synergistic effect, as groups often accomplish more than each member would alone (Edwards 1986). When the group is relatively homogeneous; that is, similar in age, sex, ethnicity, employment or residence, members are more likely to discuss experiences in greater depth than each would individually (Hawe et al 1992). A further advantage of group teaching is the relatively organized nature of the educational program. A scheduled session offers a structured time for learning, and because the session is prepared ahead of time, the topic can be more thoroughly researched and made relevant to the group's needs. A group also allows peer learning and interaction with others of relatively similar knowledge levels.

Edwards (1986) suggests that when working with groups, certain basic assumptions should be taken into account:

- Persons at all ages have the potential to learn. Individuals vary in the way they prefer to learn, and age may or may not affect the speed of learning.
- Individuals experiencing change are likely to feel stress and confusion. Some anxiety facilitates learning, but too much is detrimental. Therefore, environmental conditions should be arranged to support open exchange, problem solving, and the sharing of different ideas and values in an atmosphere of trust and acceptance.
- When students' own experiences, observations, ideas and feelings are incorporated into the teaching, they learn to clarify the beliefs and behaviours which will aid them in meeting their own learning goals.
- The depth of long term learning may depend on the extent to which the learners try to analyze, clarify or articulate experiences to others, such as family, work or social groups.
- Predisposing, reinforcing, and enabling factors influence learning.
- Active participation in the learning process enhances learning.

Groups therefore provide a challenging experience for the teacher-facilitator.

The teacher-facilitator

What makes a good group leader? Conducting group sessions is demanding, exciting and rewarding. It requires the nurse to perform many roles simultaneously: to play the organizer, leader, catalyst, participant, observer and evaluator. It is a therapeutic use of oneself to help the group achieve its goals.

Positive role modelling and strong communication skills are the most important assets for any group leader. The role which is modelled needs to be one which participants can relate to. For example, in a weight control program group, members can identify with a leader who understands the 'battle' rather than one with very extreme views, perhaps with too svelte a figure, and who may be somewhat intimidating. Depending upon the purpose of the group, a sense of fun can be a complementary asset, for people seem to learn best in a convivial atmosphere. When group sessions are enjoyable, the group tends to become more cohesive. This, in turn, promotes the interplay so important to learning. Finally, those traits which characterize the helping relationship—non-possessive warmth, genuineness and accurate empathy (Truax & Carkhuff 1967)—are of no less importance to the teaching relationship. As a group is about sharing, it is helpful if the leader is warm and sharing and encourages the same in group members. The group leader should, however, be aware of his or her own feelings, reactions, biases and values in order to be empathic while recognizing the boundaries between himself or herself and participants (Wilson 1985).

Steps in the teaching-facilitating process

Jarvis (1985) offers a five-step guide to the teaching process. The steps include: identifying the learners, identifying the topics or areas to be taught, writing learning objectives, developing the content, and evaluating the teaching plan. These steps are useful in preparing for any teaching session, particularly in the group situation.

Step 1: Identify the learners

As an initial step, characteristics of the group participants should be identified. It is important in 'pitching' the message to the audience to know members' ages, relevant cultural issues, developmental stages, educational levels, health attitudes and knowledge levels about the topic(s) to be discussed. This information can be gathered through case history notes, a formal questionnaire completed prior to the start of the group, or by informal dialogue with participants at the beginning of the first session. Informal discussion can also yield information on whether or not participants are ready to learn and what factors are affecting their motivation to learn. Learning readiness is influenced by such things as fatigue, sensory deficits, anxiety, pain and environmental distractions (Stanton 1990).

Motivation to learn is affected by many issues, including interest in the subject matter, whether or not the time of learning sessions conflicts with other responsibilities (particularly if there is a difficulty with child care), and whether or not there is social or family support for attending the group. The adult learner, having experiences to connect the teaching content to, tends to have a problem-centred orientation to learning, and is therefore usually motivated by practical application (Knowles 1980). Adults are often inclined to self-directed learning which allows time for reflection. Having time to reflect allows critical appraisal of learning and tends to foster independence of mind and action (Jarvis & Gibson 1985).

Individual differences also affect the group characteristics. Each person selectively attends to certain messages at particular times, so the 'teachable moment' varies from one learner to the next. There is, therefore, no uniformity of how the information is being received, despite the consistency of its presentation. As Egger et al (1990) suggest the message has both cause and effect, depending upon the characteristics of group members and how each is interpreting the information. Because of these individual differences, most group leaders try to discuss topics at a level which is easily understood by the majority of the group. However, it is also necessary to have an agenda flexible enough to encourage feedback, to listen to responses from group members, to clarify any issues as they arise, and to restructure elements as necessary.

Step 2: Identify the topics/areas to be taught

The subject area of group teaching is usually defined by the purpose of the group. Groups come together for many reasons, for example, to seek enrichment in their lives, to learn new skills, to share grieving, to gather support for behaviour change, to learn new strategies for self-management, and to cope with crises. It is important at the outset to clarify the purpose and expectations of the group, so that content and structure can be matched to needs. For example, those who participate in wellness groups (groups formed to discuss ways to enhance health) will expect to learn strategies to improve their quality of life and to increase their stamina and sense of well being in order to function efficiently and productively. Members of grief support groups, on the other hand, will expect to gain self-understanding, to learn strategies for coping with loss and to seek comfort.

In any group, regardless of structure, it is helpful to have an outline prepared, even if it is not strictly adhered to. At the introductory session, the leader usually attempts to lend predictability to the group by sharing the course outline, explaining her or his plans and expectations, arranging for courteous introduction of all members, describing the format of group meetings, suggesting directions the group might take, and discussing the group's duration and how it will terminate.

Step 3: Write learning objectives

Even in the most unstructured group, there are objectives which must be met. Objectives can often be negotiated with participants and should state in behavioural terms what is to be achieved by the time the group terminates or at the end of each session. Some appear below.

Example 7.1: Objectives for a group on parenting skills

By the end of the eight-week program, participants will be able to:

1. List five important concerns about parenting
2. Identify trouble spots at each developmental stage
3. Discuss eight major guidelines for effective parenting
4. Compile a list of local resources for parents
5. Identify any areas for further investigation.

Example 7.2: Objectives for a diabetes education group

By the end of the four sessions, a participant will be able to:

1. Assess his or her individual strengths and limitations in coping with diabetes
2. Discuss strategies for improving his or her self-management of diabetes
3. Demonstrate accurate calculation and administration of required medication or blood glucose monitoring
4. Complete a food plan for a one-week period
5. Identify at least one source of emotional support for the following three-month period.

It should be evident from these examples, that objectives lend structure to group work. In the same way that expected outcomes provide a template for a nursing care plan (see Ch. 4), learning objectives guide the conduct of health education groups. It is important to note that objectives are written in specific behavioural terms with defined time frames, and are oriented to the learner or participant. A behaviour is expected from the participant, something which he or she will do or discuss or perform within a stated period of time. When objectives are couched in these terms, the group leader has a master plan, or strategy for the group, and can evaluate at the end of the session or the program, whether objectives have been met and therefore whether the purpose of the group has been fulfilled.

Step 4: Develop the content

The content of most programs or sessions is developed to correspond to the objectives. If the group is a self-help group, or one which has a relatively unstructured format, the participants will provide most of the content, and the group leader will usually provide resource materials, such as books, and sources of further information and assistance. For groups such as the diabetes education group in the example above, content development may include collecting printed materials and audiovisual aids from the local diabetes association, drafting a teaching guide or 'script' for each session, preparing blank food plans for participants, reproducing informative articles for distribution to group members, and assembling teaching kits for administration of medication.

The content must be adapted to fit the group members, and to interface with existing service programs and service sites (Anderson & McFarlane 1988). Teaching materials and techniques can then be creatively developed and tailored to the needs of the group, then 'marketed' in a socially and culturally appropriate way.

Many people respond to graphically illustrated information, particularly those whose culture embodies a great deal of symbolism. Many of the health promotion materials aimed at Australian Aborigines use Aboriginal drawings to provide the identification with Aboriginal culture. Similarly, an effective teaching tool has been developed for Canadian Aborigines as part of the Native Diabetes Program in Toronto. The 'Nanabush and the Pale Stranger' story uses a cultural metaphor to present information on food, medicine and exercise to members of the Ojibway Indians. The health education message is couched in recognizable folklore and traditions of the native culture, rendering it appropriate for teaching in native communities (Hagey & Buller 1983). Bushy (1992, p. 17) cautions that it is essential to understand each culture's traditions, suggesting that nurses must be 'astutely sensitive to the fact that when scientific knowledge is presented so that it appears incompatible with a client's traditional beliefs, the traditional way will probably be accepted'.

Smitherman (1981) suggests that proper sequencing of health education content is an important aspect in conducting learning sessions. She recommends that information progress from the known to the unknown, that material which is anxiety provoking be presented first to defuse any emotional barriers, and that routine or general information be dealt with before variations and specific details. Knopke and Diekelmann (1981) add that material should be presented in such a way as to encourage critical thinking and debate, with the group leader intervening only to facilitate problem solving. These authors also advise that the group leader facilitate termination of the group. This includes encouraging and accepting expression of feelings and reminiscence, and allowing distancing devices, regression and final separation.

Lancaster (1988) offers a list of 'do's' and 'don'ts' for effective communication in teaching which are helpful in either individual or group situations.

Do:
- watch for learner clues that the message is unclear
- rephrase the message, repeat the content and ask for feedback until you are certain the learner has received the intended message
- be familiar and comfortable with the content before attempting to teach it
- speak the learner's language
- be specific when giving information
- stick to the point and be brief
- place key points up front
- be careful in teasing and joking with clients.

Don't:
- be afraid to ask questions to teach you the terms with which clients are comfortable
- be condescending—clients quickly pick up such an attitude and resent it
- allow language to alienate you from the learner.

Step 5: Evaluate the teaching plan

The method for evaluating a program's success should be devised at the time the learning objectives are developed. The success of a group can be evaluated according to both process and outcome, much like Phases 7, 8 and 9 of the Precede-Proceed model. Process evaluation addresses whether the group was acceptable or not, how many people participated, and to what extent they participated. This information is usually gleaned from compiling attendance data and participants' comments throughout the program, and by questioning members of the group in a summary evaluation at the group's concluding meeting.

Outcome evaluation attempts to determine whether the goals and objectives of the program were met. This can be done by written questionnaire or by soliciting comments in an informal way. A written questionnaire before and after the program allows an accurate estimation of group members' post-course knowledge and attitudes in relation to previously identified needs. Such evaluative information can be useful as a guide to revising a program for the future, to provide feedback to the group leader on his or her teaching strengths or weaknesses, or to judge the viability of conducting further groups.

THE ROLE OF THE NURSE IN HEALTH EDUCATION AND PROMOTION

According to Eng et al (1992) determinants of health related behaviour change are embedded in community relationships and interactions which increase community competence and enable collective mediation, negotiation and empowerment. The nurse's role in health education and promotion is thus one of interacting as a partner in health care, acting as a catalyst for change by enabling and facilitating informed choice (Kort 1987). The role of an enabler is to impart information without expectations or judgement, functioning as a health resource rather than an expert. The facilitator acts as a support for lifestyle change. Furthermore, health promotion should always be undertaken with a clear understanding of the issue of responsibility. Kort (1987) suggests that as nurses we are not responsible *for* clients or for what they do with advice and information provided by us. We are responsible *to* them—for the quality of our practice and teaching.

Community health nurses have always played a large role in health promotion, particularly as proponents of the growing trend toward healthier lifestyles. As a credible source of information, the nurse providing advice and gentle confrontation serves to reinforce large-scale efforts to promote public health. The benefits are now becoming apparent. Throughout the developed world, quit-smoking campaigns have had many positive results including an increasing number of 'quitters' and enactment of legislation banning tobacco sponsorship from sporting events. Nutrition promotion and awareness programs have also had powerful effects on consumer behaviour, as witnessed in the advertising and consumption of healthy foods. Physical fitness has also become a growing trend and there is heightened awareness of the perils of sexually transmitted diseases and drink driving. Health and healthy lifestyles are marketable commodities which can be encouraged through example, advocacy, access and information. It is therefore imperative that community health nurses continue to tap into the resources and techniques available to them, incorporating the promotion of public health into the broad spectrum of community health nursing practice.

SUMMARY

'Human behaviour is largely dependent on the nature and quality of information existing in the environment' (Labonte & Penfold 1981, p. 4). The key to effecting behaviour change is therefore the provision of appropriate information which will be of some help to those seeking change in their lives or their environment. Health education and health promotion are within the domain of most health professionals. However, it is the community health nurse who is often available and ideally situated to be the agent of change. Acceptance of, and commitment to the change agent role demands continuing efforts to keep abreast of the strategies and tactics of the teaching-learning process, and always being alert to the ways in which change can be organized around cultural, social, economic and environmental constraints and facilitating factors.

Study exercises

1. Discuss Green and Kreuter's (1991) definition of health promotion (p. 159) in relation to the principles of primary health care.

2. Using the Precede-Proceed model, devise a plan for promoting health in a mining community.
3. Discuss the criticism that many media-based health promotion programs have tended to 'blame the victim'.
4. Devise a set of learning objectives for a 'families of AIDS victims' group. Identify some of the issues which you would anticipate will be of particular concern to this group.
5. Devise a set of learning objectives for a 'migrant women's health' support group. Identify some of the issues which you would anticipate will be of particular concern to this group.

REFERENCES

Adelson P, Irwig L, Turnbull D 1992 Who attends screening mammography? Australian Journal of Public Health 16(1): 66-71
Anderson E, McFarlane J (eds) 1988 Community as client: application of the nursing process. Lippincott, Philadelphia
Baum F, Brown V 1989 Healthy Cities (Australia) Project: issues of evaluation for the new public health. Community Health Studies XIII(2):140-149
Baum F, Traynor M, Brice G 1992 Healthy Cities: the Noarlunga experience. In: Gardner H (ed) Health policy: development, implementation and evaluation in Australia. Churchill Livingstone, Melbourne pp 337-360
Borland R, Owen N, Hocking B 1991 Changes in smoking behaviour after a total workplace smoking ban. Australian Journal of Public Health 15(2):130-134
Brown V 1992 Health care policies, health policies or policies for health. In: Gardner H (ed) Health policy: development, implementation and evaluation in Australia. Churchill Livingstone, Melbourne pp, 91-117
Burnley I 1991 Stomach cancer mortality in NSW and Sydney. Australian Journal of Public Health 15(2):88-100
Bushy A 1992 Cultural considerations for primary health care: where do self-care and folk medicine fit in? Holistic Nursing Practice 6(3):10-18
Clarke K, Knowles S 1990 The drinksafe campaign, 1988-1990: a review of campaign survey data. Health Department of Western Australia, Perth
Connell R, Dowsett G, Rodden P, Davis M, Watson L, Baxter D 1991 Social class, gay men and AIDS prevention. Australian Journal of Public Health 15(3):178-189
Dignan M, Carr P 1987 Program planning for health education and health promotion. Lea & Febiger, Philadelphia
Donnelly N, Oldenburg B, Quine S, Macaskill P, Flaherty B, Spooner C, Lyle D 1992 Changes in reported drug prevalence among New South Wales secondary school students, 1983 to 1989. Australian Journal of Public Health 16(1):50-57
Edwards L 1986 Health education. In: Edelman C, Mandle C (eds) Health promotion throughout the lifespan. C V Mosby, St Louis
Egger G, Fitzgerald W, Frape G, Monaem A, Rubinstein P, Tyler C, Mackay B 1983 Results of a large scale media anti-smoking campaign in Australia: the North Coast Healthy Lifestyle Program. British Medical Journal 287:1125-1187
Egger G, Spark R, Lawson J 1990 Health promotion strategies & methods. McGraw-Hill, Sydney
Eng E, Salmon M, Mullan F 1992 Community empowerment: the critical case for primary health care. Family Community Health 15(1):1-12
English J, Hicks B 1992 A systems-in-transition paradigm for healthy communities. Canadian Journal of Public Health 83(1): 61-65
Esler-McMurray A 1980 The body shop: marketing a healthy lifestyle. The Canadian Nurse 76(4):46-48
Flynn B 1992 Healthy Cities: a model of community change. Family Community Health 15(1):13-23

Green L, Kreuter M 1991 Health promotion planning: an educational and environmental approach. Mayfield Pub., Mountain View California

Hagey R, Buller E 1993 Drumming and dancing: a new rhythm in nursing care. The Canadian Nurse 79(4):28-31

Hall W, Flaherty B, Homel P 1992 The public perception of the risks and benefits of alcohol. Australian Journal of Public Health 16(1):38-42

Hawe P, Degeling P, Hall J 1992 Evaluating health promotion: a health workers guide. McLennan & Petty, Sydney

Health Department of Western Australia 1988 Drinksafe. Health Department of Western Australia, Perth

Healthy Cities Australia 1991 Healthy Cities Australia, Sydney

Hirst S, Mitchell H, Medley G 1990 An evaluation of a campaign to increase cervical cancer screening in rural Victoria. Community Health Studies XIV(3):263-268

Holman D 1992 Quantification of morbidity and mortality caused by alcohol, tobacco and illicit drugs in Western Australia 1983-1988. Health Department of Western Australia, Perth

James R, Tyler C, van Beurden E, Henrikson D 1989 Implementing a public cholesterol screening campaign: the North Coast experience. Community Health Studies XIII(2):130-138

James R, van Beurden E, Steiner C, Tyler C, Fardon K 1990 The role of community educators in achieving Australian health goals: a public health approach to weight control on the North Coast, NSW. Community Health Studies XIV (2):146-152

Jarvis L (ed) 1985 Community health nursing: keeping the public healthy, 2nd edn. F A Davis, Philadelphia

Jarvis P, Gibson S 1985 The teacher-practitioner in nursing, midwifery and health visiting. Croom Helm, London

Knopke H, Diekelmann N 1981 Approaches to teaching primary care. C V Mosby, St Louis

Knowles M 1980 The modern practice of adult education: andragogy versus pedagogy, 2nd edn. Follet, Chicago

Kotler P 1975 Marketing for non-profit organizations. Prentice-Hall, Englewood Cliffs

Kort M 1987 Motivation: the challenge for today's health promoter. The Canadian Nurse 83(9):16-18

Labonte R, Penfold S 1981 Canadian perspectives in health promotion: a critique. Health Education April:4-9

Lancaster J 1988 Education, models and principles applied to community health nursing. In: Stanhope M, Lancaster J (eds) Community health nursing: process and practice for promoting health, 2nd edn. C V Mosby, St Louis, pp 182-209

Lasater T, Carleton R, LeFebvre R 1988 The Pawtucket heart health program: utilizing community resources for primary prevention. Rhode Island Medical Journal 71:63-67

Maccoby N, Solomon D 1981 The Stanford community studies in heart disease prevention. In: Rice R, Paisley W (eds) Public communication campaigns. Sage, Beverley Hills

McAlister A 1981 Anti-smoking campaigns: progress in developing effective communications. In: Rice R, Paisley W (eds) Public communication campaigns. Sage, Beverley Hills

McMichael A 1989 Coronary heart disease: interplay between changing concepts of aetiology, risk distribution, and social strategies for prevention. Community Health Studies XIII(1):5-13

McPherson P 1992 Health for all Australians. In: Gardner H (ed) Health policy: development, implementation and evaluation in Australia, pp 119-135

Milio N 1981 Promoting health through public policy. F A Davis, Philadelphia

Nutbeam D, Catford J 1987 The Welsh heart program evaluation strategy: progress, plans and possibilities. Health promotion, 2(1):5-18

Raeburn J, Beaglehole R 1989 Health promotion: can it redress the health effects of social disadvantage? Community Health Studies XIII(3):289-293

Schofield M, Tripodi D, Girgis A, Sanson-Fisher R 1991 Solar protection issues for schools: policy, practice and recommendations. Australian Journal of Public Health 15(2):135-141

Smitherman C 1981 Nursing actions for health promotion. F A Davis, Philadelphia

Stanton M 1990 Health education. In: B Bullough, V Bullough (eds) Nursing in the community. C V Mosby, St Louis, pp 105-127

Turnbull D, Irwig L, Adelson P 1991 A randomised trial of invitations to attend for screening mammography. Australian Journal of Public Health 15(1):33-36

Truax C, Carkhuff R 1967 Toward effective counseling and psychotherapy: training and practice. Aldine, Chicago

Wallerstein N 1992 Powerlessness, empowerment, and health: implications for health promotion programs. American Journal of Health Promotion 6(3):197-205

WHO-Health and Welfare Canada-CPHA 1986 Ottawa Charter for Health Promotion. Canadian Journal of Public Health 77(12):425-430

Wilson M 1985 Group theory/process for nursing practice. Prentice-Hall, Englewood Cliffs

Wintemute G 1992 From research to public policy: the prevention of motor vehicle injuries, childhood drownings, and firearm violence. American Journal of Health Promotion 6(6):451-464

8. The research process

Nursing research has finally come of age. In the past, research was considered the domain of nurse academics or scientists knowlegeable about statistics and computations and very much removed from nursing practice environments. The image is changing however, and research has a new look. It has become a collaborative effort between practising nurses, those in the academic setting, and multidisciplinary consultants and resource people. Today, nursing research is within the grasp of most nurses who are interested in joining a research team and curious enough to devote some time and energy to either questioning the basis for nursing practice or studying the issues and realities of practice. The following discussion provides a rationale for research in community health nursing and identifies some of the questions which need to be addressed in order to expand our knowledge base and some of the methodological approaches which can be taken to address them.

WHY RESEARCH?

Research, according to Fleshman (1985), is 'a way of thinking about problems' (p. 182). It is a structured process of asking questions, then setting out systematically to find answers. Research is therefore about understanding and explaining—about knowing (Wadsworth 1984). Knowledge is not only the discovery of new facts but also the discovery or examination of new relationships (Hockey 1991). For example, historical research attempts to disentangle the events of the time, and to shed new light on those events by the discovery of relationships. Descriptive research, as the name implies, is aimed at describing phenomena, situations and events in rich detail and thus is well suited to studies of clinical practice. Experimental research, in which a situation is manipulated by introducing variables, has important explanatory value; for example, comparing outcomes (healing, comfort) of varying treatments such as heat (a variable), soaks (another variable) and a combination of both. A further type of research, action research, describes the processes leading to planned change by carefully documenting all aspects of a situation in relation to the outcome (Hockey 1991). For example, researching the type of health promotion interventions described in Chapter 7 in relation to their outcomes, could be called action research. Smith and Hope (1992) suggest that all of the types of research mentioned above may also be considered under the umbrella of social research. Social research is well suited to investigating the social issues, practices and phenomena which interact in any given community. It is defined as 'that research which concerns itself with questions related to the interdependent interactions of members of communities and which can only be undertaken interactively with those members' (Smith & Hope 1992, p. 2).

The main reason for research in nursing is therefore to improve practice; to develop, refine and extend the scientific body of knowledge fundamental to nursing practice (Polit & Hungler 1989). A further reason for nursing research, according to these authors, is to help define the parameters of nursing, identifying the unique role that nursing has in the delivery of health care. In other words, nursing research aims to establish scientifically defensible reasons for nursing activities (Hockey 1991). In doing so, nursing research attempts to document the social relevance and efficacy of nursing practices to consumers of health care, administrators of health care facilities, insurers and government agencies. Research studies also enable nurses to share with one another by describing characteristics of nursing situations, explaining phenomena relevant to planning nursing care, predicting the probable outcomes of care giving decisions, controlling undesired outcomes and initiating activities which would rationally be expected to achieve favourable outcomes. Furthermore, nursing research attempts to develop a theoretical basis to guide practice (Polit & Hungler 1989). Nursing research therefore informs practice by verifying and expanding nursing knowledge.

THE PROCESS OF RESEARCH

Most research studies progress in a defined sequence somewhat like the following. First, an assessment is carried out. A question is posed, and literature related to the question is reviewed with a view toward substantiating, clarifying or lending perspective to the question. Second, a plan for addressing the question is conceived and developed. The plan is then systematically implemented, and the findings are analyzed. The entire process is evaluated and the information learned is shared with colleagues and the community. Finally, action is taken based on recommendations which evolved from the study. The research process is therefore a parallel and complementary adjunct to the nursing process. Both are exercises in problem solving. While the nursing process is aimed at solving care giving problems, research strives to explain the scientific foundations of practice, to understand regularities and to predict future circumstances (Polit & Hungler 1989).

In the community, there are many researchable questions which would add to our knowledge base or verify known and accepted practice strategies. Some of these were mentioned previously (in Chs 5 and 7). The discussion to follow addresses several additional areas for research investigation in an attempt to encourage community health nurses in all settings and situations to contribute to the veracity of practice by researching primary health care issues.

QUESTIONS FOR INVESTIGATION

Flynn (1988) suggests that the tenets of primary health care pose many researchable nursing questions. She categorizes these into issues which revolve around four major themes: accessibility of health services, community involvement, appropriate technology and a multisectoral approach to health care. Let us take a look at each of these areas separately.

Accessibility of health care

The issue of access to health care refers to the extent to which community health nursing services reach those who need them the most. Research questions which address these issues include:

- Which health care consumers use what nursing services?
- What are the health care needs of non-users compared to users?
- What barriers to services exist—such as cost, transportation, time and location?

Community involvement

Primary health care philosophy proposes community-care giver collaboration in health care. As the community is to be a partner in decisions which effect health care services, questions which need to be answered include:

- What is the level of community involvement in health decision making?
- What are the mechanisms for community collaboration?
- Are nursing services more widely used if community members are involved in needs assessment and planning of services?

Appropriate technology

Flynn (1988) quotes the American National Science Foundation's definition of appropriate technologies as: 'those which are decentralized, require low capital investment, conserve natural resources, are managed by users and are in harmony with the environment' (p. 176). Questions of appropriate technologies therefore address the cost effectiveness and appropriateness of health care services. Such questions include:

- How cost effective are community health nursing services as compared to similar services by other care givers?
- Are services affordable and acceptable to consumers?
- Are family home visits as effective as working with families in groups?
- Are non-professionals, such as community health workers, providing effective community health services or aspects of them?

- What are effective management and educational strategies for non-professional health workers?

Multisectoral approach

A multisectoral approach to health care encourages the team efforts of a wide range of agencies, departments and individuals in order to utilize available resources and to ensure that the input of all sectors impacting on health are considered. Questions begging investigation by all sectors include:

- What mechanisms exist in the community to promote collaboration between health care providers and the education, environment, industry and housing sectors?
- Are community-wide concerns represented by the different sectors on committees and task forces?
- What are the gaps in efforts across sectors?

In addition to these general questions, research interests and priorities are usually tied to the issues which affect a particular community, and the interests of the nurse. For example, nurses who encounter a high incidence of child abuse often begin to frame research questions around child abuse issues. Many of these questions revolve around primary, secondary and tertiary levels of prevention. For example, a study investigating the effects of antenatal classes on parenting outcomes, addresses a primary prevention issue. Comparing two different educational strategies (media vs individual teaching) for smoking cessation provides a useful basis to guide secondary prevention efforts, and an investigation of the efficacy of a nurse instigated peer support group for cancer sufferers provides insight into the effectiveness of a tertiary prevention strategy.

Many research studies are devised in response to professional need. Several authors suggest that because of a lack of conceptual clarity, nurses must begin to work towards community health nursing theory development (Hamilton & Bush 1988, Robinson 1985, Twinn 1991). Hamilton and Bush discuss approaches which would either attempt to validate existing theory in community health nursing settings or try to generate organizing frameworks from practice. For example, they identify the need for research which would identify the client of community health nursing practice. 'Without a delimitation of client focus, community health nursing theory development will continue to encompass (1) clients *in* communities, (2) clients *influenced by* communities, as well as (3) clients *as* communities' (Hamilton & Bush 1988, p. 149).

Whall and Fawcett (1991) discuss the need for studies which describe, explain, and predict family health. They suggest that nursing research of families examines the responses of families and family members to various states of health and to expected and unexpected life transitions. Family research is also necessary to test theories of the effects of nursing on family members and families and to formulate theories of predictors of family outcomes (Whall & Fawcett 1991). As mentioned in Chapter 6, this type of research is particularly needed in the area of separating families as, to date, there are very few guidelines or frameworks for nurses working with and counselling the separating family.

METHODS FOR COMMUNITY HEALTH NURSING RESEARCH

Because the community health nursing practice arena is so diverse and includes both geo-politically and ideologically defined communities, multiple theoretical and methodological research approaches must be taken (Strasser 1989). Depending upon the specific objective(s) of the study, the researcher may choose either a quantitative or qualitative method of conducting the research. These are both major and complementary approaches to nursing research and share a similar purpose: to develop nursing knowledge.

The quantitative approach assumes a positivist view of the world. Research studies begin with observations, then apply a deductive process to generate and test theory (Field & Morse 1985). Such research relies on controlled experiments, hypothesis testing, measurement and statistics. Results of studies from within this research approach have shown what nursing is about and how improvements can be made to practice not only in terms of higher standards of care, but in quality of life and cost effectiveness (Bennett 1991).

Qualitative research simply refers to any research that produces findings not arrived at by means of statistical procedures or other means of quantification. Qualitative approaches develop nursing theory inductively from the data, then test those theories in a limited way. The qualitative approach includes research about persons' lives, stories, behaviour, organizational functioning, social movements, or interactional relationships (Strauss & Corbin 1990). Although there may be quantitative elements in a qualitative study, it becomes qualitative by virtue of its analytic techniques, which are non-mathematical (Strauss & Corbin 1990). Strasser (1989) suggests that qualitative studies of communities are helpful in 'locating at-risk groups, in describing health beliefs, life styles and practices, in exploring the meanings of health, disease, and illness for the community, and in discovering what and who the community is' (p. 96). In this way, qualitative studies contribute to the goal of cultural sensitivity, allowing community members to explain culturally related issues from their own perspective (Strasser 1989). This type of knowledge is, in turn, invaluable to nursing care which is planned in collaboration with the community.

In response to Hamilton and Bush's (1988) call for theory development Streubert (1991) suggests a phenomenologic approach for community health nursing research. Phenomenology is a qualitative method of research whereby the researcher attempts to interpret people's perceptions of the world as it appears (Streubert 1991). Participants in the research describe their 'lived' experiences and the researcher attempts to identify the essence of what is revealed in order to understand the phenomena. Robinson (1985) and Streubert (1991) suggest that it would be useful for example, for community health nurses to study the phenomena of health. Phenomenology would be the likely method of choice in this case, although qualitative methods also include ethnography (an anthropological approach whereby the researcher attempts to describe a culture or aspects of a culture) and grounded theory (a process of generating theory from systematically collected and analyzed data). All three qualitative methods rely heavily on skilled observation and intensive interviewing combined with systematic detailed recording and simultaneous processing of data.

The objective of a research study thus determines its methodological approach. Duffy (1992) distinguishes between health promotion research which addresses 'the general health of the population and the development of that population to its fullest potential' and disease prevention research which investigates 'factors specific to a particular illness, disability or condition and the interventions necessary to prevent the problem' (p. 312). Hamilton and Bush (1988) suggest that there is much to be learned from research which observes and measures ways in which community health nursing structure responds to changes in political, social, economic, and legal factors, particularly when such research includes international comparisons. This type of research typically uses methods which examine patterns of health and illness; that is, the methods of epidemiology.

EPIDEMIOLOGY

Epidemiology is the study of the frequency, distribution and determinants of health and illness; the patterns of disease occurrence in human populations and the factors which influence these patterns. When a health condition occurs in a population in excess of normal expectation, it is described as an *epidemic*. At expected levels, it is considered to be *endemic* in that population. The objective of any epidemiological study is to carefully research the factors, conditions and issues related to an epidemic in order to devise strategies for control or eradication of the epidemic. In this respect, epidemiology is *applied* (rather than basic) research.

The epidemiological study may adopt an experimental approach, wherein a research question is posed and an hypothesis generated to guide investigation. Alternatively, a health problem may be identified, and the investigation may take the format of a retrospective study. Either approach requires a knowledge of the community being studied, and a holistic perspective of the individual in the context of time, place (the environment) and group membership. In addition, the investigator must be cognizant of the scientific principles relating to health and illness; the cause and course of infectious and chronic diseases; physical, biological, chemical and psychosocial factors which impact on health conditions; the art and science of nursing; consumer needs, risks and preferences; and the organization of health services. Within the lexicon of epidemiological research the history and extent of the problem to be researched is paramount. Compiling the history is accomplished by a combination of literature search, interviews and historical reports. The history traces events leading up to, then following on from the identification of the epidemic. In this respect, the investigation may be *retrospective* (taking a backward look) or *prospective* (documenting events as they occur) or a combination of both. The extent of the problem includes its geographic distribution, the proportion of the population affected, its effects on that population and the existence of time relationships or trends involved.

Medical, social, demographic, economic and political trends are very important in an epidemiological study, as they provide the context in which the problem has occurred. Throughout history, social movements have had enormous impact on epidemics. For example, current social movements, such as the environmental movement have a profound impact on public awareness and sensitivity to the global risk of malnutrition. However, one of the challenges of epidemiological research lies in the simultaneous consideration of many variables which affect states of health and illness. Mosley (1991) suggests that a key element in evaluating epidemiological studies is the concept of social synergy; that is, how one or more social factors may combine to either precipitate or alleviate a condition in society. Using the example of declining infant and child mortality rates in Kenya over the past 20 years, he explains that a variable such as women's education (a social determinant) can operate to influence infant mortality through intermediate variables (understanding disease causation, being able to meet the nutritional needs of both mother and infant). The synergystic effect of educating women, particularly in developing countries, has been shown to produce very marked improvements in child survival, to an even greater extent than medical techniques, which are often attributed with improvements in health status (Mosley 1991). Such a conclusion is only possible through systematic, epidemiological investigations which are broad enough in scope to include all elements which impact on a community's health status.

The process of epidemiological investigation is guided by conceptual models, the most commonly known of which is called the epidemiological triangle, or triad.

The epidemiological triad model

The epidemiological triad configures health and illness as a composite of three equivalent factors: the agent, host and environment. The agent is the perpetrator of disease; the host is the population at risk of contracting the disease; and the environment includes the physical, social and biological factors which surround and influence both the agent and host. Health and illness conditions can be understood by examining the characteristics and interactions between the three factors (Selby 1988).

When the usual or 'normal' pattern of health and illness prevails in a community, the epidemiological triad is seen to be in equilibrium.

Disequilibrium occurs when the pattern is altered by a disease process (the agent) or the community's response to the process (the host), or changing environmental circumstances (Selby 1988). A variation of the epidemiological triad is the epidemiological dyad in which the agent is considered as part of the environment.

The epidemiological triad has historically been used to explain infectious diseases, although epidemiological studies also seek to explore and explain non-infections conditions, such as asthma and patterns of health and wellness. However, since the global AIDS epidemic, infectious epidemics are once again becoming a focus of attention. The AIDS epidemic is thus used in the discussion that follows to illustrate the process of investigation using the epidemiological triad model (see Fig. 8.1).

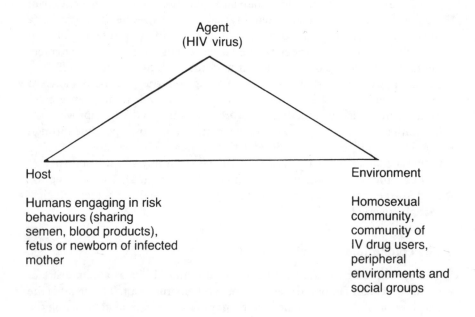

Fig. 8.1 The epidemiological triad.

The agent

The agent in a triad may be physical, such as noise or radiation; chemical, such as asbestos, pesticides or toxic waste; biological, such as a virus or bacteria; the absence of a substance (a nutritional or metabolic deficiency); or a combination of any or all of these (Stephens 1985). In the case of an infectious disease, four aspects of the agent need to be investigated: identity, natural habitat, transmission and mode of multiplication.

Our first step in an investigation of AIDS, would be to identify the causative agent, the HIV virus. Next, we would investigate the agent's natural habitat or reservoir, and its mode of escape. Reservoirs can be human, animal or environmental. The AIDS reservoir is assumed to be human (Gallo & Streicher 1987). Having gained this information, we would seek to identify the transmission of the agent from the reservoir to the host. This can be direct, for example, through intimate contact or indirect.

When an agent is transmitted indirectly, it can be vehicle borne, vector borne or airborne. Vehicles include milk (responsible for transmitting diptheria); food (the salmonella vehicle); or inanimate objects such as fomites. Vectors include arthropods which transmit African Sleeping Sickness; fleas, which have been responsible for plagues; or lice (typhus). Airborne agents can travel in dust, such as coccidiomycosis or droplet nuclei which transmit the tubercle bacillus responsible for tuberculosis (Stephens 1985). The AIDS virus is transmitted directly by semen, contaminated blood or blood products, or perinatally from infected mothers to their fetuses or newborns (Hardy & Curran 1987, Flaskerud 1992).

Another aspect which needs to be considered is the agent's mode of entry into the host. This could be via inhalation (with influenza), ingestion (with salmonella), or through the transfer of body fluids, such as occurs with AIDS. Finally, we would study the agent's multiplication in the host; whether it has multiplied with no apparent effect on the host, or to the extent of causing an infection to occur.

The host

Many factors influence a host's susceptibility to disease. The most important of these is immunity of the host. Other characteristics influencing host susceptibility to disease include nutritional status, the individual's physical and psychological state, social factors such as the presence or absence of support systems, and demographic factors (Stephens 1985). Nutritional and general physical health status has a profound effect on the development of any disease. With AIDS, for example, malnourishment may cause or aggravate the profound immunosuppression, which predisposes the AIDS victim to multiple opportunistic infections and malignancies (Flaskerud 1992). Susceptibility to the disease is also influenced by the individual's psychological state and coping ability, which are also crucial in dealing with the emotional crises accompanying the diagnosis of AIDS (Beaufoy et al 1988). Recent AIDS research also suggests a link with heavy alcohol consumption, which places an individual at risk for infections of many types (Penkower et al 1991). However, it is also noted that heavy drinkers tend to engage in more high-risk behaviours (sex with more partners, more anonymous sex, failing to use condoms) leading one to conclude that the link may be predominantly psychosocial.

Flaskerud (1992) identifies two categories of co-factors which are involved in determining the pathogenesis of HIV. These include exposure co-factors and trigger co-factors. She lists the exposure co-factors as anal receptive sex, rectal douching, multiple sexual partners, presence of genital ulcers, needle and syringe sharing, use of 'shooting galleries' (group injections), frequency of injection, use of recreational drugs, receipt of Factor VIII concentrate, blood transfusions, needlestick injuries, and in utero exposure. Trigger co-factors are further categorized as *non-infectious* co-factors such as malnutrition, use of IV and recreational drugs, prescribed drugs, allergic conditions, genetics, emotional stress, age, pregnancy and gender, and *infectious* co-factors which include antigenic overload from multiple infectious diseases (STDs, soft tissue infections, bacterial endocarditis, tubercular infections) and coincident viral infection and immune suppression (cytomegalovirus, HBV, Epstein-Barr virus, herpes viruses) (Flaskerud 1992).

Host susceptibility is also influenced by the demographic distribution of a disease or epidemic. Early descriptions of the AIDS epidemic in 1980-81 focused almost exclusively on such demographic groups as male homosexuals, blacks, IV drug users and hemophiliacs; however recent research reveals a steadily increasing proportion of people with AIDS among heterosexuals who are neither black nor IV drug users (Moss 1992). This includes a large number of heterosexual male 'sex tourists' who engage in unprotected sex with HIV positive prostitutes in countries such as Thailand and Cambodia. This situation is extremely problematic in terms of limiting the spread of AIDS to Australia, as both of these countries lie in close proximity to Australia and are promoted as affordable tourist attractions.

The dangers of sex tours are being publicized within Australia; however, the host countries tend to suppress accurate figures of the extent of the epidemic to protect the tourism industry. This illustrates the impact of social, economic and political factors on an epidemic. Obviously an international incentive is the only hope for containing the epidemic so, in 1987 the WHO established a Global Program on AIDS to investigate groups at risk and to assimilate information on the epidemic. According to Lewis et al (1991), the insights gained from studying the 9-11 million adults and 1 million children who have become HIV infected since 1981 can be expected to shape the development of national AIDS prevention and control programs during the 1990s.

Environment

Environmental factors which affect the disease process can be physical, biological, chemical or social. Physical characteristics of an environment include such things as climate, natural resources and geographic location. Biological and chemical factors include the presence or absence of infectious agents, pests, pollution or environmental contaminants. The social environment is determined by many factors such as whether it is: rural or urban; crowded or isolated; law abiding or lawless; supportive or non-supportive; tolerant or intolerant.

AIDS was originally diagnosed in a specific geographic location—the US. Early analysis of population clusters affected with the disease indicated that it may have originated in central Africa, where an earlier version of the virus may have been introduced by monkeys or via intermediaries in the distant past (Gallo & Streicher 1987). According to Biggar (1987), the widespread distribution of the disease in central Africa has promoted the idea that it arose there; however, available evidence supports the idea that it is as new to Africa as it is to the US. The effect of environment on AIDS sufferers is profound. In many geographic locations, individuals who gravitate to the social environments in which the disease is prevalent have become the target of control strategies, the effectiveness of which will only be borne out in time.

The person–place–time model

In this epidemiological model, the characteristics of the person, place and time are studied. Characteristics of persons with a particular disease or condition are compared with those without the disease or condition. Next, the place or environment in which the condition occurred is considered. These environmental characteristics are then compared with characteristics of other places or locations where the disease or condition has not occurred. Finally, patterns or trends are sought in describing the time (days, weeks, months, years) in which the disease or condition has occurred (Selby 1988).

If we were to analyze AIDS using the person–place–time model, the data would be similar to that collected in using the epidemiological triad. What distinguishes one model from another is simply its approach to data collection, as the outcome usually remains the same regardless of conceptual model used.

The web of causation model

This model best illustrates the theory of multiple causation for diseases and health conditions, and has become one of the most popular models in contemporary epidemiological investigation. Health and illness are viewed as the result of complex interrelations among multiple factors, including those related to the agent, host (person), environment (place) within a specified time frame. In an epidemiological investigation, as many factors relating to the condition as possible are investigated in order to construct a web of possible interrelationships. These interrelationships are then examined to determine the most feasible points of intervention for a control program (Selby 1988).

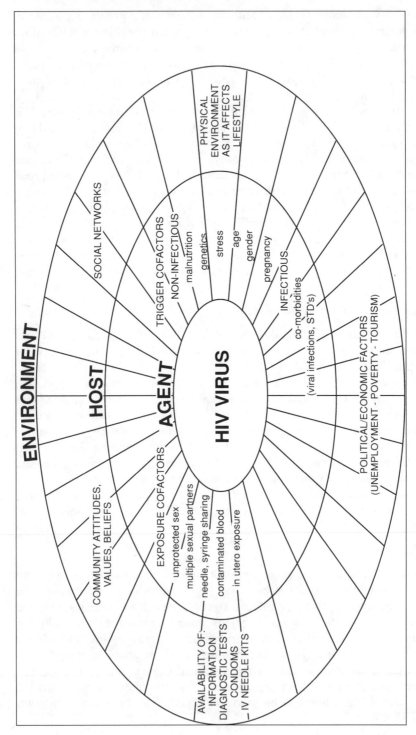

Fig. 8.2   The web of causation model, illustrating factors known to be associated with the AIDS epidemic.

A web of causation could be constructed for the AIDS epidemic to include all the factors known to be associated with the disease, as Figure 8.2 illustrates.

Epidemiological measures

As epidemiological investigation is aimed at prevention and control strategies, it is primarily observational rather than theoretical (Turner & Chavigny 1988). Data which are collected are comprised of both descriptive and substantive information (Valanis 1988).

Descriptive information is collected by observing and recording existing patterns of occurrence of health problems. Surveillance and screening programs are often major sources of descriptive data. Examining this information provides insight into the distribution of disease or health risks in a community; the types of people who are at risk of developing health problems; the conditions, disabilities or needs they have; and the services and health care providers they use for their health problems (Hood 1985).

The *substantive* contribution to the information base includes the natural history, patterns of occurrence and risk factors associated with a disease or condition (Valanis 1988). One of the initial challenges for the novice epidemiological researcher is to become familiar with the scientific language used to describe epidemiological measures. The following discussion is aimed at explaining this terminology.

Descriptive measures

Morbidity refers to the number of people in a population affected by a disease or condition. Morbidity is described in terms of incidence and prevalence. *Incidence* refers to the number of new cases of the disease or condition occurring during a specified period of time. *Prevalence* measures the amount of morbidity; that is, the total number of cases, both new and old, occurring in a population at a particular time. *Mortality* refers to the number of deaths from the illness or condition.

Rates are a mathematical measure of the frequency of a disease or condition, and provide statistical data necessary for evaluation of the health status of a group (Clark 1984). Rates are expressed as an equation which estimates the likelihood that a disease or condition would occur in a typical member of the population. Incidence and prevalence rates are those most commonly seen in epidemiological literature. *Incidence rates* measure the number of new cases of a disease or condition in a given time period.

Prevalence rates measure all cases, new and old, in a given time period. Expressed as an equation, the number of those experiencing the condition is shown as the numerator. The denominator represents the population at risk.

The *population at risk* is the total number of those in the population who are susceptible to the disease or condition, such as non-immunized children who are at risk for measles; or those with an increased potential for exposure, such as those who work in asbestos dust and are thus at risk for asbestosis (Clark 1984). This fraction is multiplied by a base number which is usually expressed as 1000 or 100 000 depending on the size of the population.

Example 8.1: Rates

$$\text{Incidence} = \frac{\text{No. of new cases in a period of time}}{\text{Population at risk during same time}} \times \text{base}$$

$$\text{Prevalence} = \frac{\text{No. of existing cases in a period of time}}{\text{Population at risk during same time}} \times \text{base}$$

Rates can be expressed as *crude rates*, which are computed for the population as a whole; *specific rates*, which can be related to certain subgroups or conditions; or *adjusted rates*, which are adjusted on the basis of such demographic characteristics as age, race or sex (Selby 1988).

Incidence and prevalence rates and other descriptive information are fundamental to planning health program priorities, utilizing resources efficiently, planning strategies to meet health needs and evaluating the effectiveness of measures used to control or prevent specific disorders (Hood 1985). However, any investigation of population health must also determine the relationship of other factors in the community to the development of disease or health conditions. For this reason, analytic measures of health must be considered.

Analytic measures

When a certain factor is suspected of having an association with the development of a disease or condition, a comparison can be made between those in the population exposed to the factor, and those not exposed to it. This is expressed as *relative risk*; a ratio of the incidence rate of those exposed and those not exposed.

Example 8.2: Risk ratio

$$\text{Relative risk} = \frac{\text{Incidence rate among those exposed}}{\text{Incidence rate among those not exposed}}$$

The relative risk ratio determines whether the rate in the exposed population is higher than in the population not exposed and, if so, by how much. If the relative risk is higher in the exposed population, the factor is identified as a *risk factor* (Selby 1988).

If there are no incidence rates available, such as in the situation where a disease or condition has already occurred and is being studied retrospectively, a risk ratio cannot be calculated. Instead, what is calculated is a mathematical ratio of the odds in favour of having the disease or condition when the factor is present, as compared to the odds in favour of having the disease or condition when it is absent. This is called the *odds ratio*.

A third analytic risk measure is called *attributable risk* or risk difference. This is the difference between incidence rates in those exposed to a disease or condition and those not exposed, and is calculated by subtracting the incidence rate in the non-exposed from the incidence rate in the exposed group (Selby 1988).

Despite the analytic tools available to assist in determining risk, caution must be taken to distinguish association from causation. Health conditions are the product of a complex web of factors: hereditary predisposition, biological characteristics, history, environmental effects, stressors and life events. For a variable to be a causative agent, five conditions must be met. First, the association between the variable and the condition or problem must be consistent and must occur in the same direction. For example, if the variable is present, the condition or problem occurs; if it is not present, the condition or problem does not occur. Second, the association must be strong. The higher the correlation between the occurrence of the variable and the problem, the greater the possibility that it is a cause and effect relationship. Third, the variable must be specific to that problem; that is, the causative variable must always produce that specific condition (for example, a rash). A fourth condition for causation concerns the time relationship. The variable must precede the problem. Fifth, the notion that the variable causes the problem must be coherent or logical in the light of known facts (Clark 1984).

In most cases a condition or problem is a result of the interconnections and interplay between many factors, some of which have combined or synergistic effects which can either shorten a latency period for developing an illness or increase its potency once it has occurred. Attributing cause is therefore a process which must be substantiated with carefully designed studies and careful analysis.

One of the most interesting (albeit confusing) epidemiological problems which reinforces the need for caution when attributing risk, concerns the link between cholesterol and cardiovascular disease. Leeder (1991) reports on a ten-year study of Welsh men which revealed that the cohort of men eating a diet *higher* in butter (and thus cholesterol) had a higher incidence of heart problems. He cautions that such findings lead one to question the relationship between 'butter eaters' and affluence, and, for example, between affluence and the disinclination to be a smoker. In calling for more epidemiological research he suggests that public health authorities have an ethical responsibility to 'carry out experiments instead of high-fibre haranguing and Reebok rhetoric' (p. 9), urging population-based studies for such prevalent issues as heart disease.

Study design

Population-based studies use three main research designs. These are described by Turner and Chavigny (1988) as:

1   The prevalence study—a cross-sectional design
2   The cohort study—a longitudinal or prospective study
3   The case-control study—a retrospective model.

The *prevalence study* describes disease distribution in a community and generates prevalence rates. For this reason, it is useful in planning nursing services to adequately meet the needs of that population, and may also serve to identify cohorts for a cohort study.

A *cohort study* collects observations for a specified length of time on two populations: an experimental group and a control group. Cumulative incidence rates are collected, and observations are made on new occurrences of a phenomenon and the factors which preceded the onset of the problem. In this respect, it is considered a prospective or forward looking study. The information collected is used to analyze risk and potential hazards, and to measure the effects of intervention for prevention and control (Turner & Chavigny 1988).

One variant of the cohort study is the *clinical trial*, where drugs or therapeutic regimens of unknown efficacy are administered to an experimental group and withheld from a control group. Clinical trials are most frequently used in such areas as cancer treatment, and are carefully monitored by ethical review committees, as mentioned in Chapter 9.

Case control studies begin with the identification of a population with a defined illness or problem, such as AIDS. A matched or comparison group is chosen for having similarities to the 'case' group in all but one respect—they do not have the illness. Each group is then asked to recall the same exposure event or lack of it, then the two groups are compared. Because the investigation backtracks from the illness or problem, this type of study is considered retrospective (Turner & Chavigny 1988).

Epidemiology in community health nursing

As is the case in conducting any research, the collaborative effort pays the largest dividends in epidemiological investigations. Most community health nurses would find the role of principal research investigator prohibitive due to time constraints and the need to maintain practice as well as research skills. Contribution to a team effort however, is manageable for many nurses once they have become familiar with the concepts, objectives and strategies of epididemiological research. Quite often, this contribution involves the organization or reorganization of data already collected in the course of practice. It may also require perusal of the literature, increased contact with other team members, re-evaluation of practice strategies, or increased social activism. Whatever the level of participation, it is important that nursing's input to the field of epidemiology be acknowledged, for it is often the nurse who, at the point of entry to health care, is able to identify the problems and issues which inhibit, maintain or enhance the world in which we and our clients live.

Despite common preparation, each nurse has a unique perspective on practice which is derived from individual experience. A nursing network remains the most valuable forum for gathering and disseminating this type of information. Research networking can be extended to the development of research consortia, groups of nurses in separate locations who collaborate in research projects. A regrettable truth in nursing is that the scientific advances made and the achievements of many members of the profession go by unnoticed or undervalued. When professional dialogue which shares successes and failures, difficulties and triumphs is promoted, the profession reaps the benefit of individual accomplishments.

SUMMARY

The practice of nursing is built upon a scientific foundation. As nursing practice has evolved, the profession has depended upon a small cadre of nurse researchers to explore and explain the theoretical underpinnings of practice and the rationality which lies at the core of practice strategies. It is now the contention of many leaders in the profession that each of us must contribute to this scientific foundation.

This chapter has provided an overview of the research approaches which are most useful to advancing nursing practice in general, and community health nursing practice in particular. There remains a great need for both basic and applied research in order to better understand communities and the people who live in them. Once we have learned the processes of systematic investigation, the key to making a research contribution lies in collegial activities, networking with others, sharing concerns and observations about our individual communities, planning strategies for investigations which would ultimately improve community health, and sharing our findings with one another and the broader community so that communities can become informed participants in attaining health.

Study exercises

1. Describe how you would devise a research study to answer the following questions in a community of your choice. Include in your plan the method, potential participants and, briefly, how you would present your findings.

    a. Which health care consumers use which nursing services?

    b. What are the mechanisms for community collaboration to help adolescents quit smoking?

    c. Are family home visits as effective as working with groups of young mothers?

2. Identify three researchable questions which would be helpful to those assisting separating families.

3. Identify the agent, host and environment variables which affect primary prevention of AIDS in adolescents. How do these variables impact on a control and prevention program?

4. What are the major issues which need to be researched before a family planning program can be instituted in a particular community? Identify a researchable question for each of these issues.

5. How would you go about researching smoking behaviour in a population subgroup (for example, young females) retrospectively, and prospectively?

6. In planning a primary prevention program for breast cancer, what research information would you need to have? Explain.

REFERENCES

Beaufoy A, Goldstone I, Riddell R 1988 AIDS: what nurses need to know. The Canadian Nurse 84(7):16-30

Bennett M 1991 Teenage mutant nurse researchers. Proceedings, First International Conference on Nursing Research: Pro-active vs Reactive. Centre for Nursing Research, Royal College of Nursing Australia, Adelaide, pp 1-12

Biggar R 1987 Epidemiology of human retrovirus and clinical conditions recognised in Haiti and central African nations of Rwanda and Gaire. In: Brader S (ed) AIDS: modern concepts and therapeutic challenges. Marcel Dekker, New York, pp 91-121

Brink P, Wood M 1983 Basic steps in planning nursing research, from question to proposal, 2nd edn. Wadsworth, Belmont

Clark M 1984 Community nursing: health care for today and tomorrow. Reston Publishing, Reston

Connolly A 1992 Redefining the AIDS risk. The Weekend Australian. Melbourne, July, 4-5 p 18

Duffy M 1992 Health promotion in the family: current findings and directives for nursing research. In: Saucier K (ed) Perspectives in family and community health. C V Mosby, St Louis, pp 311-319

Field P, Morse J 1985 Nursing research: the application of qualitative approaches. Croom Helm, London

Flaskerud J 1992 HIV disease and levels of prevention. Journal of Community Health Nursing 9(3):437-150

Fleshman R 1985 Research for community nursing. In: Archer S, Fleshman R (eds) Community health nursing, 3rd edn. Wadsworth, Monterey, pp 181-213

Flynn B 1988 Research as a guide to community health nursing practice. In: Stanhope M, Lancaster J (eds) Community health nursing, process and practice for promoting health, 2nd edn. C V Mosby, St Louis, pp 171-180

Gallo R, Streicher H 1987 Human T-Lymphotropic retroviruses (HTLV-l, ll, and lll): the biological basis of adult T-cell leukemia/lymphoma and AIDS. In: Broder S (ed) AIDS: modern concepts and therapeutic challenges. Marcel Dekker, New York, pp 1-21

Hamilton P, Bush H 1988 Theory development in community health nursing: issues and recommendations. Scholarly Inquiry for Nursing Practice 2(2):145-159

Hardy A, Curran J 1987 AIDS: a new kind of epidemic immunodeficiency. In: Broder S (ed) AIDS: modern concepts and therapeutic challenges. Marcel Dekker, New York, pp 75-90

Hockey L 1991 The nature and purpose of research. In: Cormack D (ed) The research process in nursing 2nd ed. Blackwell Scientific, London

Hood G 1985 Epidemiology. In: Jarvis L (ed) Community health nursing: keeping the public healthy. F A Davis, Philadelphia, pp 59-70

Leeder S 1991 To the heart of a slice of Caerphilly. The Australian, June 26:9

Lewis G, Finlay J, Widdus R 1991 AIDS programs in transition. World Health Forum 12:297-301

Mosley W 1991 Will primary health care reduce infant and child mortality? In: Caldwell J, Santow G (eds) Selected readings in the cultural, social and behavioural determinants of health. Health transition series No 1. Centre for epidemiology and population health. The Australian National University, Canberra pp 10-26

Moss A 1992 HIV and AIDS: management by the primary care team. Oxford University Press, Oxford

Penkower L, Dew M, Kingsley L, Becker J, Satz P, Schaerf F, Sheridan K 1991 Behavioral, health and psychosocial factors and risk for HIV infection among sexually active homosexual men: the multicenter AIDS cohort study. American Journal of Public Health 81(2):194-196

Polit D, Hungler B 1989 Nursing research: methods of appraisal and utilization 2nd edn. Lippincott, Philadelphia

Robinson J 1985 Health visiting and health. In: White R (ed) Political issues in nursing Vol 1. J Wiley & Sons, Chichester

Schipper H, Clinch J, McMurray A, Levitt M 1984 Development and validation of the functional living index cancer: FLIC. Journal of Clinical Oncology 2(5):472-483

Selby M 1988 Epidemiology, demography and research. In: Anderson E, McFarlane J (eds) Community as client: application of the nursing process. Lippincott, Philadelphia, pp 15-100

Stephens C 1985 The epidemiologic approach and methods applied to community health nursing. In: Archer S, Fleshman R (eds) Community health nursing, 3rd edn. Wadsworth, Monterey, pp 145-180

Smith D, Hope J 1992 The health professional as researcher. Issues, problems, and strategies. Social Science Press, Wentworth Falls, NSW

Strasser J 1989 Qualitative clinical nursing research when a community is the client. In: Morse J (ed) Qualitative nursing research: a contemporary dialogue. Aspen, Denver, pp 106-125

Strauss A, Corbin J 1990 Basics of qualitative research. Sage, Newbury Park

Streubert H 1991 Phenomenologic research as a theoretic initiative in community health nursing. Public Health Nursing 8(2):119-123

Turner J, Chavigny K 1988 Community health nursing: an epidemiologic perspective through the nursing process. Lippincott, Philadelphia

Twinn S 1991 Conflicting paradigms of health visiting: a continuing debate for professional practice. Journal of Advanced Nursing 16: 966-973

Valanis B 1988 The epidemiological model in community health nursing. In: Stanhope M, Lancaster J (eds) Community health nursing: process and practice for promoting health 2nd edn. C V Mosby, St Louis, pp 149-171

Wadsworth Y 1984 Do it yourself social research. Victorian Council of Social Service, Melbourne Family Care Organisation, Melbourne

Whall A, Fawcett J 1991 Family theory development in nursing: state of the science and art. F A Davis, Philadelphia

Zlotnik C 1991 Home visiting outcomes and quality of life measures. Journal of Community Health Nursing 8(4):207-214

PART 5

Into the future

INTRODUCTION

As mentioned in the opening chapter of this book, community health nurses tailor their practice strategies to the particular needs and concerns of the community. However, each community is also linked to a larger sphere of a constantly changing society which affects the way health and illness are experienced. In order to anticipate community needs within the broader societal context, the community health nurse must develop an awareness of social and political trends and issues. Such awareness allows the nurse to reflect on the community in both its immediate and potential context in order to provide a vision for the future. As community advocate, the community health nurse must therefore adopt a curious nature, exploring the meanings present in contemporary trends, examining the patterns, and anticipating the future. The chapter in this section examines a sample of trends and issues relevant to community health which, hopefully, will provoke further curiosity into the dynamic elements which are shared by even the most unique communities.

Content: Part 5

9. Trends, issues and the future

9. Trends, issues and the future

As the next century draws near, we can reflect on many changes in society, health care and nursing. The world has become a global village whose inhabitants are connected through the communications media and, for some, through population mobility. Contemporary trends can therefore be addressed from a universal perspective, rather than from the vantage point of one or another country. The discussion to follow revolves around five major issues which will affect us all as we approach the twenty-first century. These issues concern the environment, the changing face of the community, AIDS and its impact on society, ethical issues in primary health care, and the evolving role of the nurse.

THE ENVIRONMENT

The past decade has seen a proliferation of concern about the environment. Environmental issues pervade the classroom, the public press and the social consciousness of many people throughout the world. Most changes to the environment have resulted from industrial and agricultural development, and some of these changes have been advantageous. For example, in some countries there is a reduced prevalence of malnutrition and of imperfectly preserved food, provision of sufficient and uncontaminated water supplies, better housing, smaller families and increased opportunities for education (Doll 1992). However, environmental changes have also caused destruction of much natural beauty, loss of open spaces for exercise, loss of natural habitats for some species, leading, in some cases, to extinction, emission of potentially toxic chemicals into the air, and climatic alterations (Doll 1992). All of these latter changes have, to some extent, compromised health. It is now becoming acknowledged that a healthy community is one in which environmental issues are recognized as a vital element in the maintenance of health. Health must be understood in terms of ecological balance, a balance which the WHO (1989) suggests may be struck when the environment is used as a resource for improving living conditions or increasing personal well being. To achieve this balance, environmental considerations must be incorporated into healthy public policies (Labonte 1993).

Ewan et al (1992) identify the philosophical assumptions which must underpin such policies. In their opinion, decision-makers must first take responsibility for involving and supporting public participation in decisions which affect the environment. Second, the premise that human health and environment are linked must gain acceptance. Third, it must be understood that human health and ecologically sustainable development are interdependent; and fourth, equity must be considered a key component of both sustainable development and public health policy.

The commitment of many nations to these principles led representatives from 180 countries to the United Nations' Conference on Environment and Development held in Rio de Janeiro in June 1992. The conference sought to address a sobering equation for the future of the planet. Within the next 40 years, the population will almost double (from 5.5 billion to 9 billion) while the output from industrial development will probably triple (Washington Post 1992). If countries are careless about managing resources for such a future, the earth's air and water will be so polluted, the world's food supplies so diminished, and people's quality of life so compromised that the achievement of health will be untenable. The summit represented the largest environmental meeting ever held, and was about the issue of social justice; about the need for rich nations to re-assess their wasteful lifestyles and provide direct aid to Third World countries to prevent them from having to exploit their natural resources for economic survival. Despite the urgency and intensity of the situation, delegates to the Rio summit failed to reach agreement about environmental practices, primarily because of the economic imperative. In times of recession it seems domestic, rather than international, issues take precedence. Perhaps the greatest impact of the conference has been the dialogue which has been generated from the world wide publicity which surrounded it.

Schrader-Frechette (1991) advocates continued and critical discussion on the environment as a fundamental moral problem. What harms one country, harms all others. She suggests that the arguments which have polarized the issues of development vs conservation of the environment have focused on 'environmental fascism'; that is, maximizing environmental welfare at the expense of individual human good. In order to be sensitive to the full cost of planetary degradation, pollution and resource depletion, we need to re-think our environmental ethos. She recommends that a system of 'triage ethics' be instituted wherein decisions are made on the basis of the least overall harm and the fewest violations of human rights. In her view, this is the only way to secure equity across generations (Schrader-Frechette 1991).

According to Doll (1992), efforts to achieve equity must revolve around the three environmental problems of poverty, population growth, and the production of greenhouse gases. He explains that in the developing countries, as economic and educational standards rise, mortality is reduced and fertility rates fall. It is therefore imperative that the wealthy nations provide financial and educational assistance to the developing countries to help them develop culturally appropriate strategies for job creation, family planning and health maintenance.

As the largest consumers of fossil fuels and other limited resources, citizens of wealthy countries also have a responsibility to continue reducing their own fertility rates and to adopt policies aimed at reducing their production of greenhouse gases and achieving energy efficiency. Doll (1992) suggests that such policies must encourage consumers to insulate homes to avoid heat loss, substitute public for private transport, and decrease reliance on fossil fuels by using nuclear power and developing methods for obtaining energy from renewable resources (winds, tides and sun).

To be committed to primary health care mandates that preservation of the environment is considered an issue of social justice and is therefore placed on the agenda for discussion at every opportunity. At all levels, environmental issues must be dealt with collaboratively and intersectorally. Collaboration includes participating in groups aimed at heightening public awareness of the importance of preserving *all* aspects of the environment: physical, economic, cultural and social and, where possible, lobbying for the political policies which work towards preservation of the environment. Lobby groups are most effective when they include 'grass roots' citizens who care about the community, as well as nurses and other health advocates with the skills and professional networks to translate their ideas into action.

Intersectoral representation must come from the structural dimensions of a community and include members with access to public health policy making bodies (such as nurses who are members of the Public Health Association), members of the local business and political community, educationists, and representatives of a variety of cultures and minorities. This collaborative process requires 'think tank' type discussions which emerge from a global commitment to socioecological preservation, yet which generate local strategies based on knowledge of local political and economic machinations. Such an approach is reflected in the slogan 'Think globally act locally' which most recently has been adopted by the Australian Nursing Federation for their special interest group 'Nursing the Environment'. By thinking globally and acting locally, citizens of all communities will have equal input into raising awareness of the issues central to sustenance of the environment (such as poverty, nutrition, land tenure, water conservation and urbanization) and can help to ensure that they become considered as public health problems.

It is heartening to see that the Public Health Association of Australia (PHA) has attempted to demonstrate an intersectoral approach to a variety of public health issues. For example, at a national workshop on international health in February 1992, the group included discussion of the broader determinants of variability in international health status, such as international trading relationships, level of debt in poor countries, and ecosystem degradations (PHA 1992). Such an agenda is a sign of the times. Community health professionals who are caring enough to work towards health for all people, must reinforce the notion of health as a socioecological construct at every opportunity and recognize environmental issues as fundamental to securing equity, access, cultural sensitivity, and community self-empowerment.

What can nurses do?

The community health nurse can play a vital role in mediating between people and their physical, social, spiritual and cultural environment. This can be best accomplished by educating people to make informed choices related to the environment.

The nurse's first responsibility is to become self-informed, to accept the socioecological definition of health, and to seek ways of encouraging others to adopt this broader view. Where possible, nurses should join forces with others to lobby for healthy public policies which attempt to secure ecologically sustainable development. The ANF's interest group (Nursing the Environment) and public policy making bodies such as the PHA, provide an ideal forum for nurses to contribute as a unified voice. As an individual, the nurse can use the print media to make the public aware of the interrelatedness of health and the environment. This may include displaying posters and pamphlets for clients to read, and/or writing letters to the editor of local newspapers. Where possible, individual contact with local politicians helps to encourage the inclusion of nurses in any community debate on environmental issues.

At the community level, the nurse must encourage members of the community to participate in discussion on environmental issues in order to foster the notion that it is *everyone's* environment, that equity and access to physical space as well as information extends across cultures, boundaries and generations. As community advocate, the nurse can use many and varied opportunities to reinforce the necessity to recycle consumer goods, to decrease atmospheric pollution by using renewable energy (for example, solar heat) and public, instead of private, transportation.

The community health nurse can also maintain a visible presence in advocating for culturally sensitive use of the environment. This necessitates becoming familiar with the issues related to culture and land use. Strong (1990) explains that the notion of sustainability is an integral part of most indigenous cultures, and that there is much to be learned from studying indigenous people's profound relationship with their lands, as they have evolved over many centuries a 'judicious balance between their needs and those of nature' (p. 6). According to indigenous law, 'humankind can never be more than a trustee of the land, with a collective responsibility to preserve it' (Burger 1990, p. 23). Many indigenous people have utilized systems of shifting cultivation, where agricultural land was left to recover from one season's planting before it was re-seeded. However, with the growth of 'agribusiness' (large scale commercial agriculture) the old ways of protecting the land have been replaced by introducing toxic elements into the soil to hasten the growing process. Examination of such practices in relation to the struggle for returning indigenous people to their lands thus reveals that land rights is as much an environmental issue as a cultural one. Health for indigenous people will not be accomplished without maintaining their economic and mythic connections to the land. Equipped with this knowledge, the nurse can attempt to foster understanding within the community and between the groups who claim the community as their home.

THE CHANGING FACE OF THE COMMUNITY

The 'greying' of the population has been a matter of concern for some time now. With each passing year, the proportion of people over age 65 increases, and this has important implications for health care. In general, the elderly tend to utilize health care services to a greater extent than younger people because of chronic disease. Furthermore, Maglacas (1988) reports that in the industrialized countries, and increasingly in developing countries, the majority of those over 70 are women who live alone and have multiple health problems.

The rapidly rising ageing population is significant also in terms of quality of community life. Higher life expectancy and declining birth rates in many countries will ultimately result in dramatically reduced numbers of workers to support each retired person. This is problematic only in that social and economic policies have been slow to respond to such a forecast for the future. Instead, problems such as the current unemployment crisis are viewed from a technocratic individualistic ethos. Schrader-Frechette (1991) suggests that this type of approach ignores the fact that existing income distribution may be neither sustainable nor equitable in the long run, yet it is used as a basis for measuring progress. It may be useful to reconsider the ageing population issue as a stimulus for developing social policies which would capitalize on the energy, wisdom, confidence and competence of older, experienced people in helping to solve the dilemmas of youth (such as unemployment). Another avenue which should be explored is the redeployment of youth to the community services industry. Burgeoning numbers of elderly people in the population will require that an increased focus be placed on services to enhance their quality of life and maintain their functional status (Holzemer 1992). Encouraging communities to examine the interrelationships between social demographic issues which are relevant to achieving primary health care goals may be one way of promoting community self-determinism and thus community empowerment.

Unemployment is only one of a myriad of factors plaguing today's youth. Adolescent suicide and attempted suicide and other self-abusive behaviours related to low self-esteem are increasing at an alarming rate. Youth homelessness is an issue of grave concern in that it has become a revolving door syndrome, precipitated often by the same physical and psychosocial problems which are reflected in the subculture of the homeless. No definitive data exist on the number of Australian homeless youth, but the figure may be as high as 50 000 (NH&MRC 1992). These young people are prone to physical and sexual abuse, injuries and sexually transmitted diseases. They are also at risk for a range of health problems which include skin infestations, infections and musculoskeletal problems because of poor nutrition and hygiene and a lack of preventive health care (NH&MRC 1992). Some, with chronic illnesses such as asthma and diabetes are particularly at risk from a lack of access to treatment, while others fall prey to substance abuse, often engaging in prostitution to support a drug habit. For some of these young people on the drugs and prostitution treadmill, the sexual confusion which results is almost impossible to overcome. In addition, many young girls become pregnant and have babies who are, in turn, brought into an environment at risk for physical abuse and neglect.

The NH&MRC (1992) suggests that in order to confront the problems of these young people, services and information must be made available to health care workers, teachers and families. Youth health services must be planned and co-ordinated to include preventive measures, immediate treatment (such as detoxification centres) and ongoing emotional support. Primary and secondary prevention must be aimed at achieving a balance between promoting living skills and empowerment in the young, and encouraging responsibility to the family and nurturance between generations (NH&MRC 1992). A great deal of research remains to be done to investigate the effectiveness of alternative health promotion and illness prevention strategies and approaches to the problems of youth, particularly when we consider our abject failures to date. Many adolescents still engage in unprotected sex and continue to smoke, despite evidence that both of these behaviours have potentially fatal consequences.

To some extent, the problems of the young mirror the wider problems of the family in today's society. The family has evidently fallen short of providing a stabilizing counterbalance to the stresses of everyday life, for all age groups. Some of the family's problems are, in fact, societal problems. Financial pressures related to the economic recession have created a new poor; former middle class mortgagees, many of whom believed that their education and work experience would insulate them against the changing economic tides. For virtually the first time in Australian history, there is an over-supply in the professional work force, creating an unprecedented competitiveness in the marketplace. This situation has more than economic implications, as it occurs at a time when the rates of separating families are approaching 50%. The problems associated with separation and divorce exacerbate the financial strife of both parties as well as an already compromised quality of life.

The future looks equally bleak for the next generation. Parents of today are caught between competing value systems. On the one hand, they are trying to guide their children into career paths and security for the future; on the other, because of the diversity of their lifestyles, they present paradoxical role models who are having to make up the rules as they go along. Their children are becoming educated with, in many cases, higher degrees, yet face an uncertain future. Many of these young people are rejecting or delaying marriage, based on the experiences of their parents, and finding themselves approaching 30 with often materialistic values and limited preparation for caring and sharing. One could predict that if the Australian family is to survive in the future, we will have to ensure that more resources are allocated to an already overburdened family guidance and counselling system. This will not happen unless nurses become involved in research studies which identify the extent and type of trends which are emerging in practice and which heighten awareness of what some community health nurses have already identified as an urgent need for ongoing education in family counselling techniques (McMurray 1991).

Another element which has changed the face of the Australian community is the proliferation of migrants who have immigrated from many parts of the world. A multicultural society enriches the quality of life of the entire community and should build bridges of tolerance for future generations to cultivate the development of a global social conscience. However, Leeder (1992, p. 11) cautions:

> A great deal of nonsense is written and spoken about multiculturalism, as though the word were a political poultice with remarkable healing powers. The word is used as an incantation; use it often enough, and the cracks and defects in the skin of our community will heal. Instead, such repetitive use fulfils only a cosmetic function, temporarily obscuring the ageing process and the underlying realities of an intensely divided, and at times directionless society.

Leeder's thesis is that we need to identify the values which guide our definition of health and the direction we must take to allocate resources to procure health care for all. His is an important insight at a time of scarce resources; one which calls for careful exploration of 'notions of health, the right to health, equity, efficiency, and so forth, without any professional assumption that we know exactly what these values mean for the community, but with a willingness to participate critically in the debate' (Leeder 1992, p. 13). In other words, our policies must strike a balance which is culturally sensitive and yet sets clear directions for attaining health for all.

According to the Australian Bureau of Immigration, 120 000 migrants are expected to settle in Australia each year until 2031, bringing the proportion of overseas-born residents up to 24.1% by the year 2021 (Commonwealth-State Council on Non-English Speaking Background Women's Issues 1991). Many of these immigrants are refugees from war-torn countries who arrive with a special set of needs in addition to the cultural bereavement that migrants typically go through (Eisenbruch 1990). Female refugees are particularly at risk for mental stress and depression. Upon settling, the migrant family's priorities revolve around securing work for the husband and schooling for the children, while the wife remains isolated and marginalized (Commonwealth-State Council on Non-English Speaking Background Women's Issues 1991). According to this report,

Non-English Speaking Background (NESB) women experience a distinctive pattern of ill health related to their social conditions as well as to the conditions of work, once they become employed. They have higher rates of work-related illnesses and injury as well as emotional problems and, apart from Aborigines, have the least accessible and appropriate health service provision of all Australians. Authors of the report suggest that we have a responsibility to help these women, who represent 12% of the Australian female population, by heightening awareness of their plight in the workplace, the community and in the health professions; by restructuring and reforming women's occupational environment; by improving access to English language learning and interpreter services; by providing child care, torture, trauma and other rehabilitation services, and by putting policies in place for the services required (Commonwealth-State Council on Non-English Speaking Background Women's Issues 1991).

Some of these strategies, particularly in the workplace, are also appropriate for other women who often are the sole provider of the family, yet still suffer discrimination in terms of lower salaries than their male counterparts and maintain responsibility for child care. The National Women's Health Strategy has attempted to address these issues but, thus far, has been only partially implemented in some states (Commonwealth-State Council on Non-English Speaking Background Women's Issues 1991).

The health of women is very much influenced by sociocultural issues. Most women's issues revolve around women's oppression in a patriarchal society, and the choices related to liberation from that oppression. Women's right to abortion and the difficulties associated with dual homemaker and employee roles are two issues which are being discussed in a multitude of forums. Kerr (1991) suggests that the definition of women's health needs to be broadened to include more than just conditions of the uterus. She cites such important issues as osteoporosis, depression, rape, premenstrual syndrome and menopausal difficulties as areas which need to be discussed and taken seriously. By far, the most important issue in women's health is education. Swan (1992) reports that the single most effective change in health status in India has been directly related to women becoming educated. Because the nurse-client relationship is a social contract of partnership, the nurse is most often the appropriate person to provide information, health teaching, and to facilitate empowered decision making by women.

Nurses can promote women's health by becoming involved in women's networks, providing positive role models, initiating self-help groups, teaching women skills for stress management and coping, and providing the nurturing and support which many women lack in their own environment. At the political level, nurses, as a credible and numerically dominant group of women, can provide a powerful lobby for child care, reproductive rights, accessible and subsidized screening mammography, sexual health education in schools, safe and equitable working conditions for women and safeguards against medical exploitation.

The choices which inform women's decision making are legitimized by the women's movement and the consumer movement, both of which have contributed to women's knowledge of their bodies and their social possibilities (Kerr 1991). However, there is not total agreement on the contribution made to women's health and well being by the women's movement. Faludi (1992) reports that women are still at odds with the male culture they inhabit. She suggests that, throughout the last decade, there has been rising pressure by the media to halt and even reverse women's quest for equality, resulting in a backlash, or counter-assault on women's rights. She accuses the backlash rhetoric of charging feminists with all the crimes perpetuated by the media. Women are blamed for the feminization of poverty, while in every country, budget cuts have helped to impoverish millions of women and maintain pay inequities.

Faludi (1992) also charges that women are still dominated and, in some cases, financially victimized by the image consciousness perpetuated by the fashion and beauty industries, still largely controlled by males. By far her most serious allegation of victimization of women revolves around the plastic surgery industry or 'body sculpturing' as she describes it (p. 249). She cites a 1988 congressional investigation in the US which revealed 'widespread charlatanry, ill-equipped facilities, major injuries, and even deaths from botched operations' (pp. 251-252). In 1991 the dangers of breast implants finally became cause for grave public concern in many countries, including Australia, yet Faludi cites a study reported in the Annals of Plastic Surgery which had revealed as early as 1987 that the implants failed as much as 50% of the time and had to be removed (Faludi 1992).

In Australia, Faust (1992) urges caution in accepting Faludi's backlash rhetoric, declaring that Australian women have many benefits lacking in the US. These include universal health insurance, income support for single parents, maternity and paternity leave, a fairly united teaching profession within the various public services with a strong commitment to equal opportunity, an entrenched tradition of high contraceptive use backed by abortion, a solid union movement permeable to equal opportunity, sufficient respect for the women's vote to oblige both the Liberal and Labor parties to compete for it and an ineffective moral majority. Faust does not attribute all of these differences to the women's movement but suggests that 'organised feminism is too rare to support generalisations'.

Irrespective of the difficulties in measuring the gains and losses of the women's movement, women's health remains interwoven with women's status in society and, as such, must be addressed by those seeking to achieve health for all. Armstrong (1990) suggests that many maternal deaths are due to discrimination. She forwards the notion that poverty is mistakenly assumed to put everyone at equal disadvantage in health care, but reports that the highest rates of maternal death occur in societies where the status of women is lowest. She cites several studies in developing countries which revealed gender differences related to access and equity. A children's clinic in Lagos Nigeria reports that a higher proportion of boys than girls use the facility. In Bangladesh, a study found a comparable incidence of diarrhoea for girls and boys, but 66% more boys than girls were taken for treatment. In Korea, a health project found that when a cost was introduced for immunization, the population of girls dropped from equal numbers to 25% of the boys. On the Indian sub continent every sixth death of a female infant is due to neglect (Armstrong 1990). Her analysis reveals that malnourishment, underdevelopment and anemia are linked and cause maternal deaths, leading to the conclusion that there is an urgent need to raise women's status and living conditions, provide good maternity services, and educate all communities against discrimination (Armstrong 1990).

The Public Health Association of Australia argues that a prerequisite to promoting women's health would be to separate women's health issues from children's health issues (PHA 1992). Their recommendations revolve around six important health issues: sexual and reproductive health, breast feeding, education, power, aid, and violence. They cite several principles as a guide for strategy formulation which include women's right to regulate their own fertility, a de-emphasis on women as vectors of STDs and HIV infections, women's right to information related to sexuality and reproductive health, and the provision of aid in promoting choice and demystifying technologies related to reproductive health. The group, which met to discuss international health, advocated a program of awareness that violence toward women is both physical and psychological in origin. Its members suggested that empowerment of women is central to promoting health, and they identified education and access to both information and health care as the major strategies for achieving this goal (PHA 1992). In many cases, this is a role which nurses can readily adopt, particularly in the context of primary prevention programs which focus on teaching and nurturing self-reliance and self-esteem in *both* sexes while they are young.

Another group in the Australian community which is of great concern to nurses and other health professionals is the Aboriginal population. Since white settlement, Aboriginal people have never enjoyed a standard of health anywhere near that of their white counterparts. Overall, Aboriginal mortality is 2.5-3 times that of the total Australian population (Thomson & Briscoe 1992). Aborigines have a high proportion of deaths from respiratory and infectious diseases (Devaneson et al 1986). In addition, some Aboriginal groups are at high risk for AIDS. This occurs for several reasons including frequent and extensive travel between communities, a high incidence of other sexually transmitted diseases in some regions, large numbers of young people in prisons, an escalating rate of IV drug use in some urban communities and a possibility of the virus being transmitted during ceremonial activities (Torzillo & Kerr 1991).

Saggers and Gray (1991) contend that it is primarily the political economy of society which maintains inequities, however, to some extent, the health problems of Aboriginal people persist because of a lack of culturally relevant health education. Cultural relevance is fundamental to the philosophy of primary health care (Eckermann & Dowd 1992). To promote and maintain health in the Aboriginal community, it is necessary to understand the cultural context in which health messages are received. According to Gray, Trompf and Houston (1991) Aboriginal languages have no equivalent to the English word 'health'. It is therefore difficult for Aboriginal people to conceive of health as a separate aspect of their lives. This has an important implication for health teaching. Aboriginal people often interpret health issues in terms of relationships between people rather than in terms of signs and symptoms (Eckermann & Dowd 1992). In addition, many traditional Aborigines consider ill health to be a result of spirit invasion of the entire body and death is explained in terms of murder or sorcery rather than in terms of a diseased organ or a biological system breakdown (Reser 1991). Health related messages and interventions must therefore be framed in terms of culture bound beliefs. Rituals related to death and dying must also be respected. Aboriginal people believe that when people die they must be buried in their tribal land so that their spirit can be released to go to another land (Winch 1989). Arrangements must therefore be made to assist the Aboriginal community to secure the return of a deceased member who may have been hospitalized in a distant community at the time of death. Aboriginal people also prefer to have the extended family present at the time of death (Winch 1989). There are also communication protocols related to dying. For example, Menere (1992, p. 22) explains that 'the names of people who have passed away, or "finished" (the word "died" is not appreciated) should not be spoken'.

Another aspect of the traditional Aboriginal belief system relates to the concept of 'self'. Aboriginal culture revolves around the collective and thus is much less individualistic than white society (Reser 1991). A wider sense of family pervades Aboriginal society, and the family extends to those who may not be blood relations but are nonetheless classified as relations. Gray, Trompf and Houston (1991) suggest that these classificatory relationships govern almost all social interactions, including marriage.

One of the difficulties facing nurses in Aboriginal communities concerns the Aboriginal person's perspective of the nurse-client relationship. In many cases, nurses are frustrated in their attempts to encourage self-care in Aboriginal clients when the relationship is viewed by the Aboriginal as one of *provider* of care rather than of *partner* in care. According to Eckermann and Dowd (1992) turning to a health professional for help from the Aboriginal's perspective, makes the health professional responsible for all that happens, and often leads to blame and conflict when things do not go according to plan. Health teaching must therefore be couched in terms which have meaning to the family network and state the nurse's expectations very clearly. The health educator must 'tell the story' to all ages and both sexes as they see themselves within their extended family group. This includes being sensitive to the intimacy rules regulating female and male contact. In

Aboriginal society 'women's business and men's business are discrete and segregated modes of discourse and activity upheld by strict social rules' (Mobbs 1991, p. 317). For example, there is shame attached to a reproductive examination of a woman by a male doctor or nurse.

For most Aboriginal people, child rearing practices are somewhat different than in white families. Child bearing is highly valued, resulting in large families who often live in crowded conditions. Diseases which affect the capacity of women to bear children (gonorrhoea and chlamydia) have serious social impact (Gray, Trompf & Houston 1991). Mothers tend to breast feed their babies for long periods and tend to be lenient by Anglo-Saxon standards when it comes to disciplining their children (Hamilton 1981). The social problems which Aboriginal families encounter are defined by the media as physical well being, substance abuse, delinquency, domestic violence, AIDS and Aboriginal deaths in custody. However, Reser (1991) suggests that to help Aboriginal people one must also be mindful of underlying and neglected issues and concerns which include indigenous health practices, the cultural context of Aboriginal emotional experience and expression, family and kinship dynamics and support systems, and adolescent conflicts and adjustment problems. To this list, one could also add the lack of employment and educational opportunities which confronts many adolescent Aborigines. Many of these issues and concerns were identified recently in the process of investigating the issue of Aboriginal deaths in custody (Johnston 1991).

A Royal Commission was established in 1987 to examine the issues surrounding the fact that between 1980 and 1989, 99 Aboriginal and Torres Strait Islander people died in the custody of prison, police or juvenile detention institutions. The commission reported that 'in many cases death was contributed to by system failure or absence of due care' (Johnston 1991, p. 3). The importance of the Royal Commission, according to the report, lies in the fact that 'the whole range of societal and historical factors which impact on Aboriginal lives came into focus from the investigations' (Johnston 1991, p. 5). The recommendations of the report included a call for primary health care to be used as a framework for care and for the education of personnel to better serve the needs of the Aboriginal community. Other recommendations included relevant education, cultural awareness, research, resources and the input of Aboriginal people in decisions which affect their life and health. These recommendations from such a large and legitimate body, have been welcomed by health professionals and others attempting to achieve social justice, equity and access for Aboriginals throughout the Australian community and in other countries where similar problems exist.

What can nurses do?

One of the most important skills which community health nurses must possess is the ability to accurately assess a community's needs, including assessment of changing social and demographic patterns. It is therefore imperative that nurses read widely from the popular as well as the professional press and use their knowledge to stimulate change at both the policy and the grass-roots level.

Some of the strategies which nurses can engage in include bringing old people together with young people to share ideas and potential solutions, liaising with teachers to plan self-esteem workshops for adolescents, promoting such state-wide health campaigns as the Drinksafe, Quit and Sexual Health campaigns, and devising or participating in innovative programs and community support projects. One such project developed in 1992 was called 'Operation Employ Youth', an undertaking spearheaded in Western Australia by a local doctor concerned about youth unemployment and determined to network his concerns through the health professional and business community. This type of activity enhances public awareness of the health implications of social problems such as youth poverty and unemployment.

In these times of changing family structures and functions, nurses must also re-orient some of their activities to encompass family issues. With 1994 having been declared as International Year of the Family, the time is right to embark on nursing research into family issues, to upgrade family counselling skills, to initiate or extend parenting classes, and to help families devise innovative schemes for self-help.

Nurses must also become better informed about working with many cultures in a community. This is important in all settings, but particularly in occupational health, where the nurse must mediate between employers and employees, and help to interpret health needs in their cultural context. Women must also be nurtured towards empowerment by strong lobbying for consumer-driven services such as screening mammography and cervical screening. The nurse must also become visible to female politicians who may be advocates for such improvements to women's health as Medicare supported mammography or programs to aid victims of domestic violence.

In any community, the nurse must become aware of what constitutes culturally relevant health education. It is important to recognize that Aboriginal people are influenced more by their need for social cohesion than individualism, thus messages should be tailored towards extended family relationships rather than individuals. The nurse should also become aware of the Aborigines' relationship with the land and understand that 'mother earth' is the centre of their universe, the core of their culture, the origin of their identity as people (Burger 1990). Understanding the nuances of different cultural and generational groups within a community can then be imparted to others in the community in such a way as to encourage respect and mutual co-operation.

AIDS AND ITS IMPACT ON SOCIETY

One of the major primary health care goals for nurses in the upcoming decades will be to deal with the escalating prevalence of AIDS in the community. In the early stages of the epidemic, AIDS was considered to be primarily the concern of those in specialized hospital-based medical services; however, it is now considered a chronic disease and one which requires extensive community and home support (Siegel & Krauss 1991, Moss 1992). According to Mahler (1988, p. xxi) 'the fight against AIDS is a fight for health', and the fight for health lies in primary health care. The initial challenge in combatting the epidemic will be to shift people's perceptions of AIDS to a public health, rather than a moral issue. This can be best accomplished by utilizing appropriate educational strategies.

Meyer (1988) suggests that information and education are fundamental to prevention, yet cautions that information also has a potential for harm if it is sensationalized, stigmatizing, horrifying or distorted. In his view, incorrect beliefs and myths may lead to denial, blame, helplessness and passivity, and this may cause feelings of confusion and vulnerability for those with AIDS.

As the health professional most accessible to communities of families, workers and schools, it is imperative that the primary health care nurse maintains constant liaison with AIDS education agencies and sources of current information related to HIV and AIDS. An intersectoral team approach is a major goal of the Australian National HIV/AIDS strategy (Commonwealth of Australia 1989).

The major objectives of the national strategy are to provide a multifaceted attack on AIDS which includes education, prevention, treatment, care and counselling, access and participation without discrimination, research and international co-operation (Commonwealth of Australia 1989). The educational strategy is aimed at increasing the community's awareness of HIV to a level where all Australians are familiar with the facts about HIV transmission and are able to assess their own risk and make decisions about long term protective behaviours, testing and counselling. In order to accomplish this, educational presentations must shift from media campaigns which feature either overly subtle messages (women should always carry condoms), or the not-so-subtle 'grim reaper' type of campaign, to more realistic approaches. One of the difficulties of health education messages which focus on communication in sexual relations (a woman insisting on a condom) is that it makes the assumption that couples communicate freely in the context of sexual relations when, in fact, the opposite is often the case. The Grim Reaper campaign, which struck fear into the hearts of most people, has been both lauded and criticised, Harcourt and Philpot (1988) are of the opinion that it had a profound effect on preventive behaviour. Their survey of prostitutes attending Sydney STD clinics showed that the percentage using condoms with all their clients had increased from 1-5% in 1985 to 70% in 1988 (following the campaign).

Chapman (1992) suggests that health education strategies must be examined in light of current data on actual cases of HIV infection in Australia. He describes the three types of transmission (and thus risk) as follows:

• primary (first generation) involving transmission from sex between men, needle sharing, or having received HIV contaminated blood products

- secondary (second generation) involving transmission from sex with those in primary risk categories
- tertiary (third generation) involving unprotected sex with a seropositive person who is not from a primary risk group.

Chapman (1992) posits that tertiary transmission is both rare and improbable, yet is the target of most health education in Australia. He cautions that gay men not be further vilified as a victim group, but that they, and secondary risk groups (those undertaking sex tours to South-East Asia and bisexual men), be the focus of health education strategies.

Connolly (1992) reports that there has been a shift in Australia from the 1987 Grim Reaper campaign targeting the general public towards concentrating in the 1990s on the homosexual community. The Australian National Council on AIDS and its prime lobby group, the Australian Federation of AIDS organizations, still advocate general information, but many members believe that scarce resources should be deployed in getting the message to the homosexual community, particularly in light of the fact that, to date, more than 90% of AIDS sufferers in Australia have been infected through homosexual transmission (Connolly 1992). The tactic now, according to Connolly (1992), is to target the *practices* of people—first among them, sex between men. Connolly (1992) suggests that bisexual men present a particularly challenging target group in that, because they rarely frequent homosexual hangouts or read gay magazines, they are not exposed to the AIDS health education messages as often as the gay community. On the other hand, the recent decline in the rate of infection in Australia (from 3000-4500 in 1983-4 to an estimated 600 in 1989-90) suggests that homosexual men are practising safe sex more often (Connolly 1992).

Mahler (1988) advises that, to be effective, the AIDS battle requires political commitment, intersectoral action, appropriate technology and community involvement. This must be a concerted effort aimed at developing policies for action simultaneously with public education. Policies must include guidelines for employment, education, screening and testing, counselling (pre- and post-testing), income maintenance and health insurance, housing and hostels, life insurance and compensation (Commonwealth of Australia 1988). Gradually these developments are taking place with help from lobby groups and an increasing body of research which is being used to inform both the scientific and social issues surrounding AIDS (Aggleton et al 1989, Siegal & Krauss 1991, Flaskerud 1992). It is expected that as more knowledge is gained and disseminated to professionals and the public alike, HIV/AIDS victims will have greater access to new treatments and achieve an improved quality of both life and death.

What can nurses do?

The major role of community health nurses in dealing with the AIDS epidemic concerns health education. It is essential, therefore, that nurses have access to information about the disease, its co-morbidities and social implications. Because knowledge about HIV/AIDS is continually evolving it is important that the nurse maintain ongoing contact with local and national AIDS councils and the current professional literature. In addition, it is important that the nurse participate in community groups formed for either prevention of the disease or support for those already infected. Another important nursing activity concerns research into the psychological and social issues accompanying AIDS and the nursing care of AIDS victims, and disseminating the findings of such research to nursing and other professional colleagues.

Many people with AIDS are functioning members of the community and the nurse may encounter them through occupational health, family visits or school health. Nurses should seize upon opportunities for health teaching related to AIDS in the school, occupational health and community health in general, creating an awareness among members of the community that the disease cuts across all age, sex and cultural groups, and that it is clearly a public health, not a moral, issue. To do so, nurses must participate in public debate on AIDS-related issues, acting when necessary, as the mediator between various groups and the community to help overcome the stigmatization and discrimination which often accompanies the disease.

Ethical issues in primary health care

Implicit in the human rights (social justice) ethos of primary health care are certain moral and ethical issues. By far, the most important of these concerns resource allocation. Two aspects of resource allocation are relevant to social justice: balancing harms and benefits to populations, and utilizing cost-benefit analysis in decisions affecting client populations (Fry 1992). McCready (1991) explains this concern by citing the moral dilemma faced by those making resource decisions between an elderly arthritic who has been waiting three years for a hip replacement and whose taxes are used to finance an abortion for a teenager who refuses to use alternative methods of contraception. The dilemma lies in the decision to allocate greater or lesser funds to each of these cases from the common health care budget.

Many such examples exist where choices must be made for allocating resources in a way which is equitable, accessible, self-determined and culturally sensitive. Each has its ethical dilemma. For example, it is a costly exercise to preserve the life of a very ill premature infant or an equally ill elderly person in need of life-saving surgery because of the technological and professional human supports required for each. The ethical questions posed by such cases revolve around whether one family's self-determined need for a child or another's cultural beliefs related to family elders pre-empt decisions which would redeploy the resources used for each into community-based care for the mentally ill, or women's refuges, or AIDS research. The dilemma also poses the question of defining appropriate technology. What *is* appropriate technology? Who should decide? Under what circumstances?

Is this an area which should be the focus of urgent research? If so, who should allocate research funds, and from what source? Is it morally right to divert a large proportion of the research budget to AIDS research while other types of research are under-funded?

The research issue is of particular importance to nurses, in that the major bodies responsible for allocating research funds in most countries are dominated by the medical profession, and Australia's NH&MRC is no exception. Given that the medical profession's research bias is often towards *medical* rather than *health* research, one must question whether there is cause for optimism that social and cultural research may be funded which would investigate the broad questions of appropriate (rather than available) technologies, access, equity and self-determinism in health care. The issues concerned with self-determinism, adequacy of care, professional responsibility and the distribution of resources lack the high profile and kudos of high-tech medical research, because, as Robillard et al (1989) suggest, they are usually *pragmatic*, rather than *dramatic*. These issues also are a function of time and circumstances.

As client advocate, the nurse often is the health professional who must guide a client through decisions related to health care. Because of this, MacPhail (1991) suggests that all nurses must be cognizant of the ethics of advocacy. Nurses become involved in the ethics of resource allocation in the way they counsel clients towards decisions which not only affect them, but the delivery of health care to others. In the community, the nurse has multiple obligations to the individual, family, aggregate and community. He or she must decide priorities for advocacy based on either projected client outcomes, agency or public health priorities or affordability of services. For example, as client advocate for vulnerable groups such as women, migrants and the elderly, nurses often encourage lobbying for improvements to care (women's refuges, migrant health centres, elderly day care). Such improvements require a trade-off in terms of resources for other services or research which may directly or indirectly affect the same community.

Advocacy is a part of primary health care nursing and requires the nurse to have knowledge of the issues and to be able to think critically about the possible outcomes of her or his advice or suggestions. For example, a client's basic human rights includes the right to be informed, the right to be respected and the right to self-determination (MacPhail 1991). The implication is that a client also has a right to an unhealthy lifestyle or an 'at-risk' behaviour, which may cause conflict in a health professional committed to health promotion. Such a conflict may be exacerbated in the current climate of economic recession, when resources are used often unwittingly for allocative efficiency rather than on the basis of community need (Leeder 1992). According to Moccia (1992) we may have to deconstruct those systems which mediate the allocation of resources (education, legal, penal and health care systems) to allow creative solutions to be found from within communities rather than from those who seek to regulate them.

In addition to advocacy, Fry (1992) suggests that the principles of veracity, confidentiality and caring are also important in community health nursing. Veracity refers to the nurse's duty to tell the truth and not deceive the client. Confidentiality controls the disclosure of information so that clients feel that the information is safeguarded and will thus not hesitate to seek help when they need it. Caring concerns the protection, welfare or maintenance of all clients. According to Fry (1992) when all of these ethical principles are adhered to, the client gains a feeling that she or he is protected and the relationship between client, nurse and the health care system is strengthened.

Many ethical dilemmas pervade community health nursing practice, and need to be discussed as a continuing dialogue with other primary health care team members. One issue which has found its way into ethical discussions concerns the disposal of body parts. On the one hand, there is a commitment to biomedical research which may have a delayed, yet profound, impact on the community; while on the other, the family with a deceased member has the right to have all body parts returned for burial following post mortem. The family which has not been informed of removal of an organ or body part may be considered exploited at the expense of biomedical research. In the past, it was considered a prerogative of post mortem to remove body parts for research without informing the family, however, because of successful lobbying by concerned consumer groups, the family's right to choose is now on the agenda for professional discussion. As advocate for the family, the community health nurse must be aware of the responsibility to provide the family with an explanation of their rights so that family members can make informed choices related to burial.

A very different dilemma arises over the issue of AIDS testing. If mandatory HIV testing became accepted practice in the workplace as a basis for employment, it would be very difficult indeed to justify excluding those who tested HIV positive, particularly in view of the fact that as many as 50% of the results may be false positive (Aggleton et al 1989). These authors also describe the ethical dilemma related to AIDS testing for immigration and border control. They report that the Council of Europe issued a statement in 1987 that control measures at borders are scientifically and ethically unjustifiable. The Council of Europe report is backed up by a WHO report which declared that it makes little sense, in public health terms, to screen international travellers with the objective of excluding those with clinical AIDS (Aggleton et al 1989). The WHO report stated that, because of the window of uncertainty between infection and the production of antibodies, such screening would be too costly and retard only briefly the dissemination of HIV within and between countries. Despite this, a number of countries have introduced restrictions designed to deny permanent residence to those with HIV infection or AIDS (Aggleton et al 1989).

This type of ethical issue serves as a reminder that primary health care demands a global conscience; a world order with shared values, processes and structures (Perlmutter 1991). Global issues such as the Chernobyl disaster, global warming and AIDS should provoke a greater international social commitment. Perlmutter (1991) posits that nations and cultures need to be open to one another's influence, to recognize identities and diversities by accepting ethnic and religious pluralisms. He suggests that the prevailing ideology must be one of co-operation and tolerance for shared values and their varying, culturally relevant interpretations. His vision for a global civilization is thus one which is unique in a holistic sense, yet heteregeneous in nature (Perlmutter 1991).

A global commitment includes coming to terms with the responsibility of wealthy nations to allocate a proportion of their budgets to helping developing countries meet their health and educational goals. At the UNICEF summit held in 1990, it was calculated that an additional US$46 billion a year must be allocated to meet the global goals of halving malnutrition, raising the birth weight of new-born babies, and eliminating polio. The executive director of UNICEF suggested that the world must recognize that millions of lives could be saved by relying on low-cost, under-used technologies, and that the end of the Cold War should enable the redirection of billions of dollars previously wasted on armaments (Harrison 1990).

What can nurses do?

None of the ethical or moral issues in primary health care have easy solutions, yet individual nurses must come to terms with them. The most significant steps which nurses can take to prevent the exploitation of clients are to keep the issues on the agenda for discussion in all nursing forums, to practise with a sense of social responsibility and to continually examine, through research, the changing nature of health care and of the effectiveness of primary health care nursing.

Participation in area health boards ensures that nurses have a voice at such time as the budget is being discussed. Conducting research into the cost effectiveness of health care, and particularly nursing care is essential. In addition, community health nurses should spend some time reflecting on how they counsel clients in terms of their social responsibility, examining the way in which advice is given and ensuring that they are not prejudicing one family's opportunities at the expense of another's. Finally, the nurse must practise with a global conscience. In some cases, membership in such groups as Community Aid Abroad or Amnesty International casts a wider perspective on practice activities and also helps to elevate the profile of the community health nurse as a visible, socially aware participant in the community he or she is associated with.

THE EVOLVING ROLE OF THE NURSE IN PRIMARY HEALTH CARE

The major feature of primary health care is that it is responsive to the community it serves. Primary health care nursing must therefore by definition, change and evolve in conjunction with the community and society. In Australia over the past century the role of the nurse has remained relatively stable, although the context in which it is carried out has been one of continuous change (NH&MRC 1991). Changes which have affected the nursing role include the following:

- the changing role of women in society
- advances in science and technology with resultant ethico-legal dilemmas, and changing work force requirements
- changing patterns of education
- the reorientation in health care towards promotion, maintenance and self-help
- increased consumer awareness and demands for easy access to health care
- increasing economic constraints
- spiralling health care costs
- an increased proportion of aged persons, many of whom have disabilities
- a more multicultural population (NH&MRC 1991).

These changes have led to a greater need for all nurses to be aware of primary health care goals and to have a much broader based education than at any previous time in history, for according to Mahler (1985) it is nurses who hold the key to achieving health for all.

Nurses were early converts to primary health care. As mentioned in Chapter 1, the ICN and other nursing groups followed the Declaration of Alma Ata with statements of commitment to its goals and principles. Nearly a decade later, in 1987, the Australian Better Health Commission, was established to report on the health status of Australians and recommend strategies for attaining higher standards of health for the future. This group called for the development of a national primary health care policy and implementation plan to facilitate health promotion (Health Targets and Implementation [Health for All] Committee 1988). Its authors provided a moral argument for prevention by suggesting that 'The ethical and philosophical underpinning of the four broad aims of the WHO (Europe) Health For All strategy—equity in health, adding life to years (health promotion), adding health to life (reducing morbidity) and adding years to life (reducing premature mortality)—reflects a concern for maximising human potential' (p. 5). However, the report did not mention the ways in which nurses and others could work together within the framework of primary health care to achieve its aims. In 1991, the Better Health Commission released an interim report on the role of primary health care in health promotion which proposed two strategic initiatives: a national primary health care development funding program, and a set of Commonwealth state-territory agreements to provide a framework for the specific initiatives which would attempt to reorient health care and health promotion in

Australia (National Centre for Epidemiology and Population Health/National Better Health Program 1991). Although this report contained strong support for primary health care as a means to achieving health for all, it also failed to mention the important role of the nurse, emphasizing instead, the general practitioner as the key player in health promotion. However, it is expected that the profile of Australian nurses in primary health care will gradually be elevated through participation in the National Reference Centre for Continuing Education in Primary Health Care at The University of Wollongong (Howe 1992).

Despite the reports of the Better Health Commission, nurses remain the only professional group to have developed their own strategies for primary health care. In 1990, the Australian Nursing Federation (ANF) compiled a strategies document on the premise that 'nurses have the power to facilitate health for all by examining health promotion, cost effectiveness and policy over and above their role in clinical intervention' (ANF 1990, p. 3). The document lists four major factors which are recognized as fundamental in supporting the changing roles and functions of the nurse. These include nurses' attitudes and values, reorientation of education programs, better resource allocation and well-defined policies and plans for the development of nursing personnel. In order to achieve these changes the ANF calls upon educational institutions/schools of nursing, policy makers, nurse registering authorities and employing authorities to review all relevant policies and programs to reflect and incorporate the principles and values of primary health care and the health for all strategy (ANF 1990).

Attitudes and values

The most important tool which can be used to advocate for others is a sense of personal and professional worth. George and Larsen (1988) offer several methods for accomplishing this which include recognizing self-worth, valuing the contributions of colleagues, educating the public about nursing's role and capabilities, improving nursing education, rewarding initiative and creativity, recruiting non-traditional candidates into nursing, and supporting strong, effective leaders. These recommendations are highly appropriate for all nurses, but are particularly relevant for cultivating the primary health care ethos.

What can nurses do?

In accepting primary health care as the means for achieving community health, nurses must begin a professional dialogue to foster and share attitudes of tolerance for all variations of social life, particularly related to family and alternative lifestyles. For example, nurses need to understand the traumatic effect of the AIDS epidemic on the homosexual population, the difficulties of separate parenting, and the obstacles faced by women living in a patriarchal world and Aborigines living with discrimination. Nurses must also encourage respect for the migrant population, and serve as a role model for a culturally sensitive society by encouraging cultural maintenance. This involves promoting the integration of migrants in the community by learning about their respective cultures, and teaching the young to listen with tolerance to the contributions which other cultures make to society. As politically aware members of society, nurses must also have a voice against the social ills which precipitate poverty and homelessness. Every act of tolerance and advocacy can be seen as a form of political activism. To be politically active means using sound judgement, taking a stand, voicing an opinion and being a concerned citizen. Each of these are activities which normalize the social accountability of the nursing role.

Reorientation of education programs

Expansion and extension of the nurse's role to encompass primary health care requires a broad, generalist base of knowledge and skills which are continually updated and augmented by continuing personal and professional education. Community health nurses participating in the author's research into the development of expertise revealed that they are heavily influenced by both life experiences and professional experiences (McMurray 1991). It is therefore important to stress to nurses during their formal education that they must be receptive to *all* experiences in order to capitalize on experience as a means towards developing expertise.

The ANF (1990) identifies several strategies for reorienting education programs. These include lobbying governments, educational providers and employers to ensure the provision of formal award and continuing education programs which prepare for primary health care practice, as well as monitoring the content of such programs. They suggest encouraging curriculum developers and educators to ensure that primary health care is the central focus of all preregistration nurse education programs and that curriculum content includes content and experiences which will foster skills for providing primary health care. Content should include writing, using and influencing media, advocacy, political activism and lobbying, consulting and collaborating, transcultural care, enhancing self-care, research and evaluation, computer literacy and public speaking. Field experiences should also emphasize primary health care and take account of the diverse cultural context within which nurses practise, and where possible, provide opportunities for inderdisciplinary education in primary health care (ANF 1990). In addition, nurses must be encouraged to network: to join professional and interdisciplinary organizations, to publicize strategies for primary health care, to take time to be reflective and creative, then to share their ideas with one another.

For the nurse engaged in primary health care nursing, the need for ongoing education and discussion is particularly acute. Until recently, primary health care philosophy, concepts and strategies have not been a part of preservice nursing education. However, Anderson (1993) reports that this is changing. In a survey of nursing curricula she found that a majority of programs in Australian schools of nursing included a substantial component of primary health care.

Education for primary health care must be addressed in a planned and logical manner, in conjunction with state (or provincial) and national goals for nursing education, and must be relevant to the political and ecological world in which nurses and clients interact. In addition to biomedical issues, content must include current and relevant information on legal, ethical, social and political issues, and the communication skills to utilize such information. Reorientation of educational programs therefore involves structuring curriculum content to reflect current realities and prepare for future possibilities in a constantly changing community.

Resource allocation

Nurses can help with equitable resource allocation by participating in health policy groups such as the area health boards which are being introduced in most states of Australia. Nurses can also contribute by participating in costing nursing services, work force planning, helping to identify appropriate technologies, and lobbying for changes to health care provision. The most effective way of participating is to conduct or support nursing research projects which are practice-based and which describe the extent of nursing practice, the competencies required, and the comparative cost effectiveness of nursing care. This type of research will enable nurses and policy planners to make informed decisions about resource distribution. It will also help in planning for appropriate work force deployment, ensuring that rural and remote areas and vulnerable groups (Aborigines, women, migrants, the elderly) are not under-serviced. Practice-based research will also allow the profession to develop processes by which nurses can achieve a measure of control over their costs and budgets.

Policies and plans for development of nursing personnel

In addition to the research suggested above, the ANF (1990) suggests that nurses become involved in research aimed at measuring present and alternative health care systems, primary health care initiatives, primary health care education (perhaps through the national reference centre on continuing education for primary health care) and public participation in health care. One of the most important initiatives for developing nursing personnel has come from the nurse practitioner review conducted by the New South Wales Health Department. In 1991, the chief nursing officer established a task force to examine the role and function of independent nurse practitioners (New South Wales Health Department 1992). The discussion document produced by the group may be the genesis of a national movement to better utilize the nurse in the community. Its recommendations include urging endorsement and accreditation of the role of the nurse practitioner, examining the efficiency and viability of a schedule of selected rebateable services for accredited nurse practitioners, and exploring potential referral processes and relevant changes to legislation to facilitate the practice of nurse practitioners in the provision of health services (New South Wales Health Department 1992). The report is cause for optimism that the role of the nurse in independent or relatively autonomous practice will gain the recognition it deserves. It may provide the impetus for discussion of a system whereby independent nurse practitioners can provide to this over-burdened, expensive and impersonal health care system an equitable, accessible, cost effective, and user-friendly means of achieving health and caring in the community.

SUMMARY

Community health nursing is on the threshold of an exciting era. The world has become a kaleidoscopic macrocosm of communities which influence and are influenced by one another's history, culture, goals and commitments. Several contemporary trends and issues of this global society impact on the practice of community health nursing. These include recognition of the importance of the environment in relation to health, changing patterns and trends in families, communities, and society, the impact of the AIDS epidemic, and the evolving role of the nurse in helping to meet the needs of diverse and ever-changing populations.

Each of these trends is of consequence to the future of community health nursing. Nurses must develop a global conscience, and become involved in efforts to sustain the population and preserve the environment. In order to function as advocates for the community, nurses must become economically, politically and culturally aware of the social, as well as biomedical, issues which impact upon families and their individual members. Empowerment and tolerance must be fostered within the community's subcultures as well as in the community itself. To achieve this, the community health nurse must adopt a visible profile within the community ecosystem; one which suggests a partnership for self-determined health care. This must begin with educational processes which are relevant to role requirements and which continue to evolve with the needs of the community. Finally, community health nurses must seek to galvanize all members of the profession into action, to examine, research and publicly debate their role in securing no less than health and caring for all people.

Study exercises

---

1. List four specific cultural practices which directly affect health in a migrant group in your community.
2. Identify one activity which would demonstrate your ability to 'think globally, act locally'.

3. Describe how you would go about promoting the health of homeless youth.
4. Critically analyze Leeder's statement on p. 207 that multiculturalism obscures the underlying realities of a directionless society.
5. Identify the major constraints to overcoming discrimination against females in developing countries and discuss ways in which nurses can help to counter these.
6. Discuss the ethical dilemmas related to counselling a family of low socioeconomic status who wish to enter an IVF program.
7. Discuss the issue of redeploying health education resources to primary and secondary, rather than tertiary, risk groups in the case of HIV infection.

REFERENCES

Aggleton P, Homans H, Mojsa J, Watson S, Watney S 1989 AIDS: scientific and social issues. Churchill Livingstone, Edinburgh
Anderson D 1993 Primary health care and pre-registration nursing education: the Australian perspective. Unpublished Masters thesis, The Flinders University of South Australia, Adelaide
Armstrong S 1990 Labour of death. New Scientist 125(1710):32-37
Australian Nursing Federation 1990 Primary health care in Australia: strategies for nursing action. ANF, Melbourne
Burger J 1990 The GAIA atlas of first peoples. GAIA Books, London
Chapman S 1992 Dogma disputed: potential endemic heterosexual transmission of human immunodeficiency virus in Australia. Australian Journal of Public Health 16(2):128-144
Commonwealth of Australia 1988 AIDS: a time to care a time to act: towards a strategy for Australia. Australian Government Publishing Service, Canberra
Commonwealth of Australia 1989 National HIV/AIDS strategy. Australian Government Publishing Service, Canberra
Commonwealth-State Council on Non-English Speaking Background Women's Issues 1991 The national non-English speaking background women's health strategy. Australian Government Publishing Service, Canberra
Connolly A 1992 Redefining the AIDS risk. The Weekend Australian, Melbourne, July 4-5 p 18
Devaneson D, Furber M, Hampton D, Honari M, Kininmonth W, Peach H 1986 Health indicators in the Northern Territory. Northern Territory Department of Health, Darwin
Doll R 1992 Health and the environment in the 1990s. Australian Journal of Public Health 82(7):933-941
Eckermann A, Dowd T 1992 Strengthening the role of primary health care in health promotion by bridging cultures in Aboriginal health. Australian Journal of Advanced Nursing 9(2):16-20
Eisenbruch M 1990 The role of cultural bereavement in health transition in a multicultural society. In: Caldwell J, Findley S, Caldwell P, Santow G, Cosford W, Braid J, Broers-Freeman D (eds) What we know about health transition. The Health Transition Centre, The Australian National University, Canberra, pp 644-656
Ewan C, Young A, Bryant E, Calvert D 1992 National framework for health impact assessment in environmental impact assessment Vol 2. University of Wollongong, Wollongong
Faludi S 1992 Backlash: the undeclared war against women. Chatto & Windus, London
Faust B 1992 Backlash wallows in feminist backwater. The Australian, Melbourne, July 8:19
Flaskerud J 1992 HIV disease and levels of prevention. Journal of Community Health Nursing 9(3):137-150

Fry S 1992 Ethics in community health nursing practice. In: Stanhope M, Lancaster J (eds) Community health nursing: process and practice for promoting health 3rd edn. C V Mosby St Louis, pp 69-89

George T, Larsen J 1988 The culture of nursing. In: Baumgart A, Larsen J (eds) Canadian nursing faces the future. C V Mosby, Toronto, pp 63-74

Gray A, Trompf P, Houston S 1991 The decline and rise of Aboriginal families. In: Reid J, Trompf P (eds) The health of Aboriginal Australia. Harcourt Brace Jovanovich, Sydney, pp 80-122

Hamilton A 1981 Nature and nurture. Aboriginal child rearing in central Arnem Land. Australian Institute for Aboriginal Services, Canberra

Harcourt C, Philpot R 1988 On the Grim Reaper campaign. The Medical Journal of Australia, 149:162-163

Harrison M 1990 World summit on children. Family Matters 27:12

Health Targets and Implementation (Health for All) Committee 1988 Health for all Australians. Australian Government Publishing Service, Canberra

Holzemer W 1992 Linking primary health care and self-care through case management. International Nursing Review 39(3):83-89

Howe B 1992 News release. Minister's Office, Commonwealth Department of Health, Housing and Community Services, Canberra

Johnston E 1991 National report, Royal Commission into Aboriginal Deaths in Custody. Australian Government Publishing Service, Canberra

Kerr J 1991 Nursing and feminism. In: J Kerr, J MacPhail (eds) Canadian nursing: issues and perspectives 2nd edn. pp 62-67

Labonte R 1993 A holosphere of healthy and sustainable communities. Australian Journal of Public Health 17(1):4-12

Leeder S 1992 Valuable health: what do we want, and how do we get it? Sidney Sax Oration, Australian Journal of Public Health 16(1):6-14

McCready D 1991 Don't copy Canada's health care system. Policy Options, October:8-10

McMurray A 1991 Expertise in community health nursing. Unpublished doctoral thesis, Department of Education, University of Western Australia, Perth

MacPhail J 1991 Ethical issues and dilemmas in nursing practice. In: J Kerr, J MacPhail (eds) Canadian nursing; issues and dilemmas 2nd edn. pp 198-208

Maglacas A 1988 Health for all: nursing's role. Nursing Outlook 36(2):66-71

Mahler H 1985 Nurses lead the way. WHO press release, Geneva

Mahler H 1988 Opening address, World Summit of Ministers of Health on Programs for AIDS Prevention. WHO, UK Government, London, 26-28 Jan. x-xiv

Menere R 1992 Remote area nursing orientation manual. Faculty of Health Sciences, University of New England, Lismore

Meyer A 1988 Introduction, World Summit of Ministers of Health on Programs for AIDS Prevention. WHO, UK Government, London, 26-28 Jan., pp 23-28.

Mobbs R 1991 In sickness and health: the sociocultural context of Aboriginal well being, illness and healing. In: Reid J, Trompf P (eds) The health of Aboriginal Australia. Harcourt Brace Jovanovich, Sydney, pp 292-325

Moccia P 1992 In 1992 A nurse in every school. Nursing & Health Care 13(1):14-18

Moss A 1992 HIV and AIDS: management by the primary care team. Oxford University Press, Oxford

National Centre for Epidemiology and Population Health/National Better Health Program 1991 The role of primary health care in health promotion in Australia. Australian Government Publishing Service, Canberra

National Health and Medical Research Council 1991 The role of the nurse in Australia. Australian Government Publishing Service, Canberra

National Health and Medical Research Council 1992 Health needs of homeless youth. Australian Government Publishing Service, Canberra

New South Wales Health Department, Nursing Branch 1992. Nurse practitioners in New South Wales, a discussion paper. New South Wales Health Department, Sydney

Perlmutter H 1991 On the rocky road to the first global civilization. Human Relations 44 (9):897-920

Public Health Association of Australia 1992 Workshop on international health. PHA, Canberra

Reser J 1991 Aboriginal mental health: conflicting cultural perspectives. In: Reid J, Trompf P
    (eds) The health of Aboriginal Australia. Harcourt Brace Jovanovich, Sydney, pp 218-291
Robillard H, High D, Sebastian J, Pisaneschi J, Perritt L, Mahler D 1989 Ethical issues in
    primary care: a survey of practitioners' perceptions. Journal of Community Health
    14(1):9-17
Saggers S, Gray D 1991 Aboriginal health and society. Allen & Unwin, Sydney
Schrader-Frechette K 1991 Ethics and the environment. World Health Forum 12:311-321
Siegel K, Krauss B 1991 Living with HIV infection: adaptive tasks of seropositive gay men.
    Journal of Health and Social Behavior 32(Mar):17-32
Strong M 1990 Forward. In: J Burger The GAIA atlas of first peoples. GAIA Books,
    London
Swan N 1992 Health: a tale of two centuries. Annual Research and Development Lecture,
    Edith Cowan University, Perth
Thomson N, Briscoe N 1992 Overview of Aboriginal health status in Western Australia.
    Australian Government Publishing Service, Canberra
Torzillo P, Kerr C 1991 Contemporary issues in Aboriginal public health. In: Reid J,
    Trompf P (eds) The health of Aboriginal Australia. Harcourt Brace Jovanovich Sydney,
    pp 216-380
Washington Post 1992 What Rio is all about. Editorial, June 2, Washington
Winch J 1989 Why is health care for Aborigines so ineffective? In: Gray G, Pratt R (eds)
    Issues in Australian nursing 2. Churchill Livingstone, Melbourne pp 53-70
WHO 1989 Environmental impact assessment: an assessment of methodological and
    substantive issues affecting human health considerations. University of London, WHO
    Report No 41, Geneva

Appendix 1: Standards for community nursing practice

Reprinted with permission of the Australian Council of Community Nursing Services (ACCNS)

STANDARD 1. The community nurse fulfils the obligations of the professional role.
STANDARD 2. The community nurse establishes and maintains enabling interactions in professional relationships.
STANDARD 3. The community nurse provides effective and holistic nursing care.

STANDARD 1

The community nurse fulfils the obligations of the professional role.

Nursing behaviours

The community nurse in any practice setting:
1.1 Complies with the profession's code of ethics
1.2 Functions in accordance with legislation and common law affecting nursing practice
1.3 Acts to protect the rights of the client
1.4 Acts to maintain the safety of the client/self/others
1.5 Acts to rectify unsafe nursing practice or professional misconduct
1.6 Practices within own abilities and qualifications
1.7 Ensures the effective management of human financial and material resources
1.8 Evaluates own practice and participates in peer review
1.9 Continually updates knowledge and skills
1.10 Participates in activities designed to maintain or improve the quality of <u>nursing care</u>
1.11 Contributes to nursing research and development of nursing knowledge
1.12 Participates in decision making about health care planning, practice, and evaluation

1.13 Fosters progress towards the goal of 'Health For All By the Year 2000' within a culturally diverse community

1.14 Participates in activities of the profession's organisations

1.15 Interprets nursing and promotes the nursing profession to the community

STANDARD 2

The community nurse establishes and maintains enabling interactions in professional relationships

Nursing behaviours

The community nurse in all professional interactions:

2.1 Uses and promotes effective communication

2.2 Conducts caring and effective interpersonal relationships

2.3 Establishes and maintains effective communication with the health team to achieve co-ordinated care

2.4 Acts as an advocate to assist individuals to make informed decisions

2.5 Creates and uses opportunities for learning

STANDARD 3

The community nurse provides effective and holistic nursing care

Nursing behaviours

The community nurse in providing nursing care in any practice setting:

3.1 Acknowledges the individual as an holistic being and the need for nursing care to reflect this belief

3.2 Recognises the individual's right to partnership and enables their active participation in nursing care

3.3 Enhances achievement of optimum self care

3.4 Identifies significant others and provides the support they require

3.5 Collects information which enables the formulation of a comprehensive written data base through assessment and from a variety of other sources

3.6 Analyses and interprets the data in order to identify the individual's:
    — health strengths and resources
    — health concerns, both actual and potential
    — expectations of care

3.7 Formulates with the individual a written plan of care which:

— addresses health strengths, concerns and expectations
— includes a statement of expected outcomes and selected nursing interventions

3.8 In collaboration with the individual implements the plan of care

3.9 Evaluates the individual's response to care, significant changes in health status and progress towards expected outcomes

3.10 Records the process of care

3.11 Formulates a written plan of care for discharge/transfer which ensures continuity of care

3.12 Evaluates the effectiveness of the process of nursing care

---

STANDARD 1

The community nurse fulfils the obligations of the professional role

Nursing behaviours

The community nurse:

1.1 Complies with the profession's code of ethics

1.1.1 recognises the client's right to autonomy

1.1.2 documents customs, religious and dietary practices which the patient wishes to maintain while receiving nursing care

1.1.3 takes steps to obtain the support needed by the patient to maintain customs, religious and dietary practices

1.1.4 addresses others with respect and uses preferred name

1.1.5 recognises the primary responsibility of nurses is to those people who require nursing care

1.1.6 maintains confidentiality of information

1.1.7 uses judgement in sharing information

1.2 Functions in accordance with legislation and common law affecting nursing practice

1.2.1 maintains current registration

1.2.2 observes registering authority legislation

1.2.3 meets legal requirements binding on registered nurses, e.g.:
— handling and storing of drugs
— reporting of child abuse
— notification of communicable diseases
— trespass

1.2.4 practises in accordance with the common law of duty of care, e.g.:
— is aware of the need to seek expert advice when assignments require knowledge or skill beyond educational preparation and/or competence
— intervenes when policies or practices may impede care or contravene the law

1.2.5 observes agency policies, programs and procedures

1.2.6 maintains legible, dated and signed nursing records

1.3 Acts to protect the rights of the client

1.3.1 supports the right of clients to make decisions about health care

1.3.2 informs the client of their rights to
- participate in decisions concerning own care
- give or withhold consent to treatment, procedures and/or participation in research programs
- refuse treatment or interview in the presence of students
- see own health record using correct administrative procedures

1.3.3 observes and protects the client's right to dignity, privacy and respect

1.3.4 seeks the client's informed consent before implementing nursing care

1.3.5 seeks the client's consent before obtaining health history from other health professional or agency

1.3.6 gives the client appropriate information

1.3.7 acts as an advocate for the client

1.3.8 informs others in the health team when the client requires additional information outside the sphere of nursing practice

1.3.9 supports the client in circumstances of unwarranted opposition, abuse, neglect or possible physical harm

1.3.10 supervises students of nursing in all practices until competence has been achieved

1.3.11 supports the client in their informed decision to terminate nursing and other health care

1.3.12 obtains interpreter services as necessary

1.4 Acts to maintain the safety of the client/self/others

1.4.1 initiates action, independently or in co-operation with others, to minimise health hazards in the environment

1.4.2 can specify employing agency policies relating to safety, e.g. fire safety, cardiopulmonary resuscitation techniques

1.4.3 complies with agency policies relating to safety

1.4.4 takes reasonable care to assure own health and safety and to avoid adversely affecting the health or safety of others

1.4.5 uses such protective clothing and equipment as is necessary to avoid illness or injury

1.5 Acts to rectify unsafe nursing practice or professional misconduct

1.5.1 serves as a positive model for peers and nursing students

1.5.2 discusses with person concerned, inappropriate professional behaviours

1.5.3 reports and documents accidents, errors, incidents or complaints

1.5.4 informs the person concerned of the action to be taken

1.5.5 follows up incidents to monitor recurrence of unsafe practice or unprofessional conduct

1.5.6 challenges inappropriate orders and decisions by nurses and other health professionals, e.g. orders for medication or treatment; illegible and unclear orders; the implementation of inappropriate orders; the withholding of treatment; orders that have the potential to harm the individual or violate their rights

1.5.7 recognises, corrects and reports own errors

1.5.8 follows employer/professional organisations' disciplinary guidelines in dealing with, documenting and reporting unsafe practices and professional misconduct of nurses and other health care workers

  1.6 Practices within own abilities and qualifications

1.6.1 recognises own knowledge and skill level

1.6.2 understands the requirements of the position description for the position sought or held

1.6.3 recognises own strengths and utilises them

1.6.4 informs employer of assignments requiring knowledge or skill beyond own level of competence

1.6.5 demonstrates knowledge of principles underlying any practice undertaken

1.6.6 when unsure seeks guidance from competent colleague

1.6.7 practices within own position description.

  1.7 Ensures the effective management of human, financial and material resources

1.7.1 works within employing agency pool

1.7.2 monitors use of resources

1.7.3 takes action as required to ensure cost effective use of resources

1.7.4 co-operates with others to maintain resources required for effective nursing care

1.7.5 co-operates with others to maintain resources in effective working order

1.7.6 sets priorities, organises and defines responsibilities of individual nurses

1.7.7 delegates nursing care assignments matching the person's needs to the nurse's capability

1.7.8 ensures nursing assignments are completed

1.7.9 provides support and feedback to assist team members achieve optimum work performance

1.7.10 takes action when resources are inadequate to meet the standards of nursing care

1.7.11 contributes towards collection of required statistical data

1.7.12 organises work distribution fairly and equitably

1.7.13 considers responsibilities and workloads of other personnel.

  1.8 Evaluates own practice and participates in peer review

1.8.1 develops personal performance goals that are congruent with position description and agency objectives

1.8.2 assumes responsibilities for self evaluation against the position description

1.8.3 checks own practice against agency policies/procedures

1.8.4 contributes to the peer review process for nursing colleagues

1.8.5 recognises and acknowledges colleagues' strengths

1.8.6 completes self evaluation and peer assessment process within agreed time frame

1.8.7 acknowledges the findings of peer review

1.8.8 implements the strategies to increase skills suggested during peer review

1.8.9 seeks learning experiences to overcome identified limitations in own performance.

1.9 Continually updates professional knowledge and skills

1.9.1 assesses personal learning needs and sets objectives for professional development

1.9.2 seeks learning experiences to achieve professional development objectives

1.9.3 attends staff development programs

1.9.4 reads current nursing journals

1.9.5 identifies and uses resources available to meet own learning needs

1.9.6 is familiar with theories, practices and advances pertaining to current nursing practice

1.9.7 seeks guidance with unfamiliar interventions

1.9.8 attends demonstrations related to new equipment or interventions

1.9.9 participates in multidisciplinary conferences

1.9.10 draws attention to literature which may have relevance to the current practice area

1.9.11 provides pertinent articles for colleagues

1.9.12 demonstrate innovative transfer of principles and practice of nursing care between practice settings

1.10 Participates in activities designed to maintain or improve the quality of nursing care

1.10.1 clarifies with the individual their expectation of care required and received

1.10.2 participates in review of nursing care

1.10.3 identifies problems in care delivery and suggests remedial action

1.10.4 co-operates with health care team members and significant others to implement remedial action to improve care

1.10.5 provides demonstration and/or supervision for learners as required

1.10.6 structures learning experiences for nursing colleagues

1.10.7 co-operates in implementing policies and programs

1.10.8 is familiar with aims and methods of quality assurance programs and co-operates in implementation of quality assurance activities.

1.11 Contributes to nursing research and development of nursing knowledge

1.11.1 adheres to ethical considerations and employing agency's guidelines to protect the individual's rights when research is being undertaken

1.11.2 initiates, participates in and/or facilitates nursing research

1.11.3 disseminates results of research through publication of work

1.11.4 draws colleagues' attention to pertinent research findings

1.11.5 provides learning resource material to facilitate understanding of nursing research and/or increase nursing knowledge

1.11.6 incorporates the findings of research into nursing practice.

1.12 Participates in decision making about health care planning, practice and evaluation

1.12.1 is informed about current health problems and community concerns

1.12.2 contributes to the development of nursing division and agency philosophy, objectives, policies, programs and procedures

1.12.3 participates in revision of guidelines for practice, procedures and nursing care delivery

1.12.4 serves on relevant committees

1.12.5 promotes co-operation among nurses and other members of the multidisciplinary health team

1.12.6 facilitates the dissemination of information from the practice area to decision makers

1.12.7 presents the nursing point of view when participating in discussions of health care issues.

1.3 Fosters progress towards the goal of 'Health For All by the Year 2000' within a culturally diverse community

1.13.1 has knowledge of WHO goal of 'Health For All by the Year 2000' (HFA 2000) and its associated definitions and programs

1.13.2 recognises that the basis of HFA 2000 strategy is primary health care

1.13.3 is able to define primary health care

1.13.4 is able to articulate the registered nurse's role in primary health care

1.13.5 initiates and/or contributes to the profession's or community's activities designed to promote health

1.13.6 acts as a positive role model for health

1.13.7 recognises the implications in the Australian context of HFA 2000 e.g. the need to:
— restate health policy to reflect equity in health and care
— re-allocate health care resources
— restructure health delivery services
— redirect educational preparation of health personnel

— respect the knowledge and skills brought by the client to the health care interaction

1.13.8 recognises that a crucial factor in the provision of effective health care is its relevance to an individual's cultural context.

1.14 Participates in activities of the professional's organisations

1.14.1 is a financial member of at least one nursing organisation

1.14.2 participates at meetings of the nursing organisation of which (s)he is a member

1.14.3 regularly attends professional organisation meetings

1.14.4 takes responsibility to be informed about nursing matters at state, national and international levels

1.14.5 acts within the professional organisation to establish and maintain equitable social and economic conditions

1.14.6 contributes to the work of the professional organisations.

1.15 Interprets nursing and promotes the nursing profession to the community

1.15.1 is familiar with the ACCNS philosophy and definitions and standards for the profession

1.15.2 informs members of the community and/or other health disciplines of the nurse's role within own practice setting

1.15.3 knows the criteria for entry into nursing.

STANDARD 2

The community nurse establishes and maintains enabling interactions in professional relationships

Nursing behaviours

The community nurse in all professional interactions with individuals and colleagues:

2.1 Uses and promotes effective communication

2.1.1 introduces self on first contact

2.1.2 addresses other by preferred name

2.1.3 makes the purpose of the communication clear

2.1.4 uses verbal and non-verbal communications that are congruent

2.1.5 uses appropriate terminology

2.1.6 confirms interpretation of communication

2.1.7 reinforces confidentiality of information

2.1.8 uses active listening skills

2.1.9 is sensitive to an individual's needs to express feelings

2.1.10 accepts the individual's right to refuse to answer personal questions

2.1.11 recognises the degree to which an individual's illness or disability may impair effective communication

2.1.12 modifies interaction on the basis of the individual's response

2.1.13 analyses the factors that influence the effectiveness of the process
— identifies strengths and weaknesses in own communication
— initiates action to improve ineffective communications
— implements appropriate methods for enhancing the strengths and limiting the weaknesses in communications

2.1.14 makes prompt, objective and accurate verbal and written reports

2.1.15 uses established channels of communication and lines of authority

2.2 Conducts caring and effective interpersonal relationships

2.2.1 acknowledges and respects people, their individual background, values, beliefs and perspective, and their consequent needs and behaviours

2.2.2 empathises with individual feelings and reactions

2.2.3 refrains from making or expressing value judgements

2.2.4 creates a climate in which each individual feels accepted and respected

2.2.5 orientates people new to a system/environment

2.2.6 utilises assertiveness skills

2.2.7 recognises own strengths and utilises them

2.2.8 acknowledges own weaknesses and endeavours to redress them

2.2.9 gives and accepts honest self-disclosure

2.2.10 provides constructive feedback

2.2.11 responds constructively to feedback

2.2.12 recognises stress in colleagues and takes appropriate action, e.g.:
— discusses with colleagues
— assists colleagues to take action
— supports colleague in informing superior

2.3 Establishes and maintains effective communication with the health team to achieve co-ordinated care

2.3.1 correctly identifies concerns for referral to appropriate personnel

2.3.2 initiates referrals to other disciplines where necessary

2.3.3 supports the individual in presenting their point of view to other health professionals

2.3.4 considers requests for assistance from other personnel

2.3.5 seeks information from other personnel where appropriate

2.3.6 familiarises self with plans formulated by other team members

2.3.7 utilises expertise of other health disciplines

2.3.8 provides adequate documentation when referring clients

2.3.9 documents involvement in group programs or activities

2.3.10 participates assertively and effectively in interdisciplinary interactions

2.3.11 allows opportunity for discussion and differing opinions

2.3.12 recognises the validity of opposing viewpoints on ethical issues

2.3.13 assists individuals to co-ordinate their health care program

2.3.14 is courteous and approachable to members of other health disciplines

2.3.15 documents client care clearly concisely and accurately.

2.4 Acts as an advocate to assist individuals to make informed decisions

2.4.1 assists the individual to identify sources of information and explore the options available

2.4.2 ensures that information on which individual decisions may be based:
— is complete
— is in comprehensible language (see 2.1.3)
— is non-judgemental
— takes account of the individual's present knowledge and understanding

2.4.3 interprets information from other members of the health team as necessary

2.4.4 identifies resources to help the individual elicit information about alternative health treatments and their consequences

2.4.5 assists the individual to take action about any aspect of health care

2.4.6 seeks additional information from appropriate sources

2.4.7 supports the individual's decisions by: e.g.:
— listening to individual's point of view
— verifying interpretation of decision and rationale for the decision
— documenting the decisions
— presenting/interpreting point of view to others
— interceding on individual's behalf with others

2.4.8 motivates and enhances client participation in self care

2.4.9 informs the client of services available from other members of the health care team.

2.5 Creates and uses opportunities for learning

2.5.1 uses opportunities for learning as they arise

2.5.2 structures learning experience

2.5.3 facilitates learning by sharing knowledge and skills

2.5.4 acknowledges the influence of 'role modelling'

2.5.5 applies principles of teaching/learning, e.g.:
— sets objectives
— assesses 'entering behaviour' and previous learning
— motivates the individual
— actively involves the individual in the learning situation
— provides opportunities for practice; feedback from the individual; feedback to the individual; reinforcement of teaching

2.5.6 proceeds from familiar to unfamiliar, simple to complex

2.5.7 uses language appropriate to the learner

2.5.8 develops a teaching outline that is realistic and has logical sequence

2.5.9 provides, or identifies resources for learning

2.5.10 refers teaching (s)he cannot do to appropriate personnel

2.5.11 identifies learning needs of new staff and works with them in devising a plan to meet those needs

2.5.12 maintains knowledge of current developments and research in professional practice.

STANDARD 3

The community nurse provides effective and holistic nursing care

Nursing behaviours

The community nurse in any practice setting:

3.1 Acknowledges the individual as an holistic being and the need for nursing care to reflect this belief

3.1.1 recognises that each individual is a unique entity who
— encompasses physical, psychological and spiritual elements
— is influenced by genetic, cultural, environmental, socio-economic and political factors

3.1.2 acknowledges the interdependence of these elements and factors and the effect of this interdependence on the individual's health

3.1.3 provides nursing care in the understanding that this care will be ineffective if all elements and factors are not taken into account throughout the process of care.

3.2 Recognises the individual's right to partnership and enables their active participation in nursing care

3.2.1 accepts that nursing care will be ineffective unless the individual's right to partnership is taken into account throughout the process of care

3.2.2 consults with the individual and enables their collaboration throughout the process of care.

3.3 Enhances achievement of optimum self care

3.3.1 encourages progressive responsibility for self care
— encourages self care to the individual's optimum ability
— provides relevant information/resources to enable self care
— promotes the individual's and/or significant other's acceptance of dependence when appropriate

3.3.2 incorporates plans for self care
— takes into account the individual's knowledge and skills, motivation and limitations of physical condition.

3.4 Identifies significant others and provides the support they require

3.4.1 consults with the individual to identify significant others

3.4.2 consults with significant others providing relevant information and identifying concerns

3.4.3 provides resources/supports necessary.

3.5 Collects information which enables formulation of a comprehensive written data base through assessment and from a variety of other sources

3.5.1 includes information about socio-economic and environmental factors, and psychological, spiritual, cultural and physical behaviours
— daily living activities
— physical assessment
— activity pattern
— home, family and employment situation
— social network and supports
— community resources utilised

3.5.2 incorporates relevant data from all sources
— individual
— significant others
— other health professionals
— existing records

3.5.3 uses a range of techniques including observation, interview, physical examination and measurement.

3.6 Analyses and interprets the data in order to identify the individual's health strengths and resources, health concerns, both actual and potential, and expectations of care

3.6.1 recognises environmental factors impacting on client health and safety

3.6.2 identifies the individual's perception of health status and expectations of care
— assesses the individual's knowledge and understanding of health concerns, perception of optimal health, reactions to previous illnesses, expectations of nursing care

3.6.3 determines individual strengths and resources, e.g.:
— knowledge and understanding
— motivation to participate in care
— skills and abilities
— significant other's involvement
— utilisation of aids and resources

3.6.4 identifies actual and potential health concerns through interpretation of the data
— analyses data

— identifies and documents the actual health concerns on the care plan

— identifies and documents the potential health concerns considered to be a high risk for the individual

3.6.5 indicates that data interpretation has been verified with the individual

— provides opportunity for individual to read assessment documentation

— validates with the individual the health concerns identified

— records the individual's agreement with the assessment

— requests the individual's permission to validate assessment with significant others.

3.7 Formulates with the individual a written plan of care which:

3.7.1 addresses health strengths, concerns and expectations

3.7.2 identifies opportunities for learning and health education

3.7.3 establishes priorities and plans for resolution or alleviation of health concerns

— identifies and takes action for health concerns that pose an immediate risk to the patient

— orders health concerns according to priority, taking account of person's perception

— validates the priority of health concerns with the individual

3.7.4 refers to other disciplines health concerns outside the scope of nursing

— collaborates in other care givers to optimise care delivery

— identifies health concerns requiring referral

— liaises with other health team members records referrals to other disciplines

3.7.5 clarifies with the client expectations for nursing care and contracts realistic parameters

3.7.6 includes a statement of expected outcomes and selected nursing interventions

3.7.7 states expected outcomes of nursing care in measurable terms which include a time frame. Expected outcomes include:

— a verb which is person orientated

— behavioural or clinical state to be achieved

— means of measurement

— conditions and time frame for achievement as contracted with the client

3.7.8 selects nursing interventions to achieve the expected outcomes

— selects interventions in accordance with current nursing knowledge and practice

— consults with nurse experts and other team members

— takes account of patient safety

— engages in discharge planning

3.7.9   establishes priorities for the implementation of nursing care
- takes account of the individual's activity patterns, preferences, appointments and social needs
- establishes with the individual the order in which care will be given

3.7.10   incorporates the care prescribed by other disciplines
- liaises with other health professionals regarding care
- clarifies unclear orders
- questions orders perceived to be inappropriate

3.7.11   determines the resources required to implement the plan
- determines level of self care
- organises the resources required
- determines the number and skill levels of nurses and other health workers required to give time
- reports any shortfall in requirements.

  3.8   In collaboration with the individual implements the plan of care

3.8.1   involves the individual in the care
- encourages individual participation in care and activities of daily living taking into account the limitation imposed by the immediate health status and therapy
- where appropriate, and with individual's consent where possible, provides information and guidance that allows significant others to participate in the care
- supports the individual in their informed decision to terminate nursing and other health care

3.8.2   maintains comfort, privacy, dignity, and safety
- addresses the individual by their preferred name
- provides for auditory and visual privacy
- safeguards the individual and others by recognising potential hazards and preventing or rectifying dangerous situations
- implements established procedures in emergency situations
- takes the individual's comfort into account when giving care
- implements the care with the individual's permission

3.8.3   applies critical thinking processes in giving care
- is able to state the rationale underlying the statement of expected outcomes and nursing interventions on the care plan and in discussion with the individual

3.8.4   ensures continuity of care
- exchanges and documents pertinent information during care
- collaborates with the individual
- maintains up-to-date care plans
- adheres to written care plans
- allocates staff to promote continuity of care
- participates in care conferences

3.8.5 maximise opportunities for health education
    — utilises opportunities for health teaching
    — implements the health education program throughout the care
    — prepared the client for self help following discharge.
  3.9 Evaluates the individual's response to care, significant changes in health status and progress towards expected outcomes
3.9.1 re-assesses the individual's health status
3.9.2 measures the actual outcomes using the means of measurement stated in the expected outcomes
3.9.3 compares actual outcomes with the expected outcomes
    — judges the degree of progress towards the expected outcomes
3.9.4 reviews with the individual the outcomes of nursing care
    — informs the individual of the actual outcomes
    — discusses the degree of progress towards the expected outcomes with the individual
    — reminds the client that discharge from nursing care will occur when mutually agreed expectations of care are met
3.9.5 communicates the findings of the evaluation to the health team
    — discusses the evaluation findings as appropriate at multidisciplinary meetings, nursing meetings, ward rounds, or on a one to one basis
3.9.6 revises the plan of care in accordance with evaluation findings
    — revises the priorities, expected outcomes of care and nursing interventions
    — resets priorities of health concerns
    — adjusts time frame/criteria for expected outcomes
    — selects nursing interventions
    — dates and signs revisions on care plan
3.9.7 consults with the individual regarding the revised plan of care
3.9.8 consults with significant others as appropriate
3.9.9 implements the revised plan of care.
  3.10 Records the process of care
3.10.1 documents health concerns
3.10.2 includes notation of priorities; details of nursing interventions; plans for health teaching and discharge planning
3.10.3 records the actual outcomes and degree of progress towards the expected outcomes
3.10.4 records revisions to the nursing care plan
3.10.5 incorporates these details into the permanent record
3.10.6 dates and signs nursing records.
  3.11 Formulates a written plan of care for discharge/transfer which ensures continuity of care
3.11.1 ensures that discharge from nursing care is understood and mutually undertaken

3.11.2 identifies the support services and resources necessary for discharge/transfer or continuing care

3.11.3 initiates referrals to relevant personnel/agencies

3.11.4 collaborates with significant others to ensure support of client after discharge

3.11.5 provides a discharge summary which includes
— the nursing care plan at discharge
— all information needed for continuity of care
— dates and times for future appointments

3.11.6 forwards copies of summaries to appropriate agencies.

3.12 Evaluates the effectiveness of the process of nursing care

3.12.1 is familiar with the aims and methods of quality assurance programs

3.12.2 participates in review of the process of nursing care

3.12.3 identifies strengths in care delivery and provides positive reinforcement

3.12.4 identifies deficits in care delivery and suggests remedial action

3.12.5 co-operates with others to implement remedial action

3.12.6 draws attention to literature which may have relevance

3.12.7 structures learning experiences for nursing colleagues

---

GLOSSARY OF TERMS

In this document 'nurse' refers to a registered nurse. (All underlined words are further defined).

ACCOUNTABILITY	The state of being answerable for one's decisions and actions. Accountability cannot be delegated
ACTUAL PROBLEMS	Those problems present at the time an assessment is made.
ASSESSMENT	(See nursing process).
CRITERION	A descriptive statement which is measurable and which reflects the intent of a standard in terms of performance, behaviour, circumstances or clinical states. A number of criteria may be developed for each standard.

DATA COLLECTION

The process of obtaining data concerning the <u>individual's</u> past and present health status and daily living patterns. Both subjective data (as described by the individual, his/her family or significant others) and objective data (as elicited by observation and examination and from records and reports) are included.

DATA INTERPRETATION

The analysis and synthesis of information gathered from and about the <u>individual</u>.

EVALUATION

The process of determining the extent to which goals/objectives have been achieved. Actual performance or quality is compared with <u>standards</u> in order to provide feedback mechanism which will facilitate continuing regulation and control.

EXPECTED OUTCOME

A statement of anticipated results of <u>nursing intervention</u> which will be observe in the individual. It may be long term, intermediate or short term and will include a <u>criterion</u> (or criteria) against which to measure the actual outcome.

HOLISTIC

This term is derived from the Greek word 'holos' (whole) and 'refers to an understanding of reality in terms of integrated wholes whose properties cannot be reduced to those of smaller units' (Capra 1983). In relation to nursing care, holism implies that each person must be regarded as a single entity encompassing components of mind and body which are interconnected and interdependent.

An extension of this concept envisages each person as a part of a larger whole, and as acting interdependently with a specific physical and social environment.

Capra, F (1983) <u>The Turning Point</u> Bantam, New York.

INDIVIDUAL

Refers to the person who is the consumer of nursing care. The term can be used interchangeably, where appropriate, with the words 'groups' or 'community' to designate two or more people who are the collective consumers of nursing care.

NURSING AUDIT

A formal detailed systematic review of records in order to evaluate the quality of nursing care by comparing the documented evidence with accepted standards of criteria. Nursing audit may be undertaken retrospectively or concurrently.

NURSING CARE PLAN

A written statement of the individual's problems, expected outcomes and prescribed nursing intervention.

NURSING DIAGNOSIS

A statement of actual/potential problems based on individual needs that require nursing intervention in order to be resolved.

NURSING HISTORY

A record of information collected by the nurse when interviewing the individual or his significant others.

NURSING INTERVENTION

Specific nursing activities carried out by the nurse for and on behalf of the individual.

NURSING PROCESS

The application of a planned, systematic approach to nursing care. The four phases are:

Assessment—the collection and interpretation of data and the identification of the individual's health strengths, resources and concerns.

Planning—the determination of priorities, expected outcomes and nursing interventions.

Implementation—the delivery of planned nursing intervention.

Evaluation—a continuous activity which compared actual outcomes with expected outcomes and which directs modification of nursing care as required.

OUTCOME	The results of care in terms of the individual's health status. Actual performance or quality is compared with <u>standards</u> in order to provide a feedback mechanism which will facilitate continuing regulation and control.
PATIENT PROBLEM	A condition or situation arising from a need with which the <u>individual</u> requires assistance.
PEER REVIEW	The <u>evaluation</u> of performance of individuals or groups by colleagues using established <u>criteria</u>.
PHILOSOPHY	A statement of a set of values and beliefs which guides thoughts and actions.
POLICY	A definite course of action adopted by an agency.
POSITION DESCRIPTION	Details of <u>accountability, responsibility,</u> formal lines of communication, principal duties, entitlements and performance appraisal. It is a guide for an employee in a specific position within an organisation.
POSITION SPECIFICATION	Details of the attributes and qualifications required for a specific position within an organisation.
POTENTIAL PROBLEMS	One which the individual has a high risk of developing.
PRIMARY HEALTH CARE	Essential health care made universally accessible to individuals and families in the community by means acceptable to them, through their full participation and at a cost that the community and country can afford. (WHO Alma-Ata 1978).
PRIMARY NURSING	The organisation of a nursing service in which nurses are assigned to an individual so that the total care of an individual is the responsibility of one nurse, the primary nurse.

PROCESS	The activities and interactions between those providing care and the recipient of care.
QUALITY	Quality is a degree of excellence.
QUALITY ASSURANCE PROGRAM	A planned, systematic use of selected evaluation tools, designed to measure and access the structure, process and/or outcomes or practice against established standards, and the institution of appropriate action to achieve and maintain quality.
QUALITY CONTROL	The regulation of structure and process in order to ensure outcomes are consistent with established standards.
RESPONSIBILITY	The obligation that a person assumes when undertaking to carry out delegated functions. The person who authorizes the delegated function retains accountability.
SIGNIFICANT OTHER	This acknowledges the benefit of moving away from limited definition of family and relationship (as defined by the individual) is of maximum effective consequence.
STANDARD	The desired and achievable level of performance corresponding with a criterion or criteria against which actual performance is measured.
STRUCTURE	The organisational characteristics of the setting in which a service is delivered.

Appendix 2: Community assessment tool

Reprinted from Clark with permission of Appleton & Lange

I Bibliographical Data

Community Location

Where is the community located?

What are the community boundaries?

General Description

What type of community is it (i.e. rural, urban, geopolitical, emotional)?

How much area does the community cover?

What is the community population?

What type of official community government exists? How does it function? How effective is it?

Who are the prominent officials?

Who are the unofficial leaders? What leadership style do they employ? How do they derive their power?

Are there any particular political affiliations within the community (e.g., strong Republican sentiments)?

Are there any prominent topographical features in the area (i.e., lakes, rivers, mountains, railroad lines, major highways)?

What are the significant events in the community's history?

Who are significant informants in the community?

Population Characteristics

What is the age composition of the population?

What is the sex distribution in the community?

What major ethnic groups and races are represented? In what proportion? How do these groups interact? Who has power? Who does not? How is power exercised?

Are particular ethnic groups primarily new immigrants or residents of long standing?

What is the average income level for the community? How wide is the range in average family income? What portion of the community population have incomes below poverty level?

What is the prevailing educational level in the community? What is the attitude toward education?

What is the usual marital status of the population? What is the typical family configuration?

What are the major religious affiliations in the community? How do religious groups interact? What types of community service programs are offered by religious groups? How does religion impinge on health?

What is the usual employment level in the community? How does the unemployment rate compare with that of the nation? The state? Where do most residents work? Within the community or outside? What are the major industries in the area? What industries are the major employers? What are the typical occupations of community residents? What health hazards, if any, are presented by local industry?

Are there any significant patterns of population change?

Environmental Characteristics

What types of housing are available? Are most housing units owned or rented? What is the average number of persons per dwelling? What are the prevailing property values? What is the typical rent? What is the general condition of housing available? What portion of the available housing is inadequate in terms of sanitation? Safety? What health hazards, if any, are presented by area housing?

What is the source of community water supply? How are sewage, sanitation, and waste disposal handled?

What protective services are available? How adequate are they?

What is the local accident rate? What are the prevailing rates for insurance?

What transportation resources exist? How many residents own cars? What other forms of transportation exist? Are bus routes, schedules, etc., adequate for community needs. How costly is transportation? Are there major thoroughfares nearby leading to large metropolitan areas?

What educational facilities are available? What educational programs are offered? Do they provide community service programs? What educational support services are available (i.e., libraries)?

What communication network exists? What formal communications media are available? What are the informal modes of communication? What type of communication takes place with the outside world?

What recreational facilities are available? What potential health hazards do recreational facilities provide?

What nuisance factors exist in the community?

Health Status Indicators

What is the annual birth rate?

What percent of pregnancies involved prenatal care?

What percent of pregnancies were illegitimate?

What is the annual abortion rate?

What is the overall death rate?

What is the maternal death rate?

What is the infant death rate?

What is the neonatal death rate?

What are the annual rates for specific causes of death?

What are the age-specific death rate?

What are the incidence and prevalence rates for specific diseases?

How do morbidity and mortality figures compare with national/state figures?

What is the overall immunization rate?

How do these rates compare with those of previous years?

What is the general nutritional level of community residents? What marketing facilities are available? How expensive are food items? What percent of the typical family budget is spent on food? What food supplement programs are available? How well are they utilized?

What health services and resources are available? What types of health personnel are available? What types of health facilities are available? Are personnel and facilities adequate to meet community needs? Are there preventive, promotional, therapeutic, and rehabilitative services available? Are there services available to meet the needs of all age groups represented in the population? What emergency services are available? What health education programs are presented? What official and voluntary health agencies are present in the community? How far away are health services not found in the community?

What are the prevailing community attitudes toward health and health care? How are health and illness defined? Are promotive and preventive measures utilized? What folk health practices are utilized? How are health services financed? Are health programs budget priorities? What portion of the population have health insurance? How well are health services utilized?

II Analysis of Data

What health problems are perceived by the nurse?

What health problems are perceived by local residents?

What health problems are perceived by other health professionals and community leaders?

What action is currently being taken to solve these problems?

How have previous problems of a similar nature been solved?

What are the community's expectations with regard to these problems? Who should solve them? Can they be solved

Are the resources necessary to solve these problems present in the community?

APPENDIX 3: The Friedman family assessment model (short form)

Two words of caution are called for before using the following guidelines in completing family assessments. First, not all areas included below will be germane for each of the families visited. The guidelines are comprehensive and allow depth when probing is necessary. The student should not feel that every sub-area needs to be covered when the broad area of inquiry poses no problems to the family or concern to the health worker. Second, by virtue of the interdependence of the family system, one will find unavoidable redundancy. For the sake of efficiency, the assessor should try not to repeat data, but to refer the reader back to sections where this information has already been described.

IDENTIFYING DATA

1. Family name
2. Address and phone
3. Family composition
4. Type of family form
5. Cultural (ethnic) background
6. Religious identification
7. Social class status
8. Family's recreational or leisure-time activities

DEVELOPMENTAL STAGE AND HISTORY OF FAMILY

9. Family's present developmental stage
10. Extent of developmental stage fulfillment
11. Nuclear family history
12. History of family of origin of both parents

ENVIRONMENTAL DATA

13. Home characteristics
14. Characteristics of neighbourhood and larger community
15. Family's geographic mobility

16. Family's associations and transactions with community
17. Family's social support network

FAMILY STRUCTURE

18. Communication patterns
    — Extent of functional and dysfunctional communication (types of recurring patterns)
    — Extent of affective messages and how expressed
    — Characteristics of communication within family subsystems
    — Types of dysfunctional communication processes seen in family
    — Areas of closed communication
    — Familial and external variables affecting communication
19. Power structure
    — Power outcomes
    — Decision-making process
    — Power bases
    — Variables affecting power
    — Overall family power
20. Role structure
    — Formal role structure
    — Informal role structure
    — Analysis of role models (optional)
    — Variables affecting role structure
21. Family values: Compare the family to American or family's reference group values and/or identify important family values and their importance (priority) in family.
    — Congruence between family's values and values of family's subsystems as well as family's reference groups and/or wider community
    — Variables influencing family values
    — Are these values consciously or unconsciously held by the family?
    — Presence of value conflicts in family.
    — Effect of the above values and value conflicts on health status of family.

FAMILY FUNCTIONS

22. Affective function
    — Family's need-response patterns
    — Mutual nurturance, closeness, and identification
    — Separateness and connectedness
23. Socialization function

- Family child-rearing practices
- Adaptability of child-rearing practices for family's situation
- Who is (are) socializing agent(s) for child(ren)?
- Value of children in family
- Cultural beliefs that influence family's child-rearing patterns
- Social class influence on child-rearing patterns
- Estimation about whether family is at risk for child-rearing problems and if so, indication of high risk factors
- Adequacy of home environment for children's needs to play

24. Health care function
    - Family's health beliefs, values, and behaviour
    - Family's definitions of health-illness and their level of knowledge
    - Family's perceived health status and illness susceptibility
    - Family's dietary practices
    - Adequacy of family diet (recommended 24-hour food history record)
    - Function of mealtimes and attitudes toward food and mealtimes.
    - Shopping (and its planning) practices.
    - Person(s) responsible for planning, shopping, and preparation of meals
    - Sleeping and resting habits
    - Exercise and recreation practices (not covered earlier)
    - Family's drug habits
    - Family's role in self-care practices
    - Family's environmental practices
    - Medically based preventive measures (physicals, eye and hearing tests, and immunizations)
    - Dental health practices
    - Family health history (both general and specific diseases—environmentally and genetically related)
    - Health care services received
    - Feelings and perceptions regarding health services
    - Emergency health care services
    - Dental health services
    - Source of medical and dental payments
    - Logistics of receiving care

FAMILY COPING

25. Short and long-term familial stressors
26. Family's ability to respond, based on objective appraisal of stress-producing situations
27. Coping strategies utilized (present/past)
    - Differences in family members' ways of coping

— Family's inner coping strategies
— Family's external coping strategies
28. Areas/situations where family has achieved mastery
29. Dysfunctional adaptive strategies utilized (present/past)

Table B-1   Family composition form

Name (Last, First)	Gender	Relationship	Date/place of birth	Occupation	Education
1. (Father)					
2. (Mother)					
3. (Oldest child)					
4.					
5.					
6.					

Index